Ferri's BEST TEST

Second Edition

Ferri's BEST TEST

A Practical Guide to

Clinical Laboratory Medicine and Diagnostic Imaging
Second Edition

Fred F. Ferri, MD, FACP

Clinical Professor
Alpert Medical School
Brown University
Providence, Rhode Island

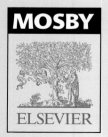

1600 John F. Kennedy Blvd.
Ste 1800
Philadelphia, PA 19103-2899

ISBN: 978-0-323-05759-2

FERRI'S BEST TEST: A PRACTICAL GUIDE TO CLINICAL LABORATORY MEDICINE
AND DIAGNOSTIC IMAGING
SECOND EDITION

Notice

Knowledge and best practice in this field are constantly changing. As new research and experience broaden our knowledge, changes in practice, treatment and drug therapy may become necessary or appropriate. Readers are advised to check the most current information provided (i) on procedures featured or (ii) by the manufacturer of each product to be administered, to verify the recommended dose or formula, the method and duration of administration, and contraindications. It is the responsibility of the practitioner, relying on their own experience and knowledge of the patient, to make diagnoses, to determine dosages and the best treatment for each individual patient, and to take all appropriate safety precautions. To the fullest extent of the law, neither the Publisher nor the Author assumes any liability for any injury and/or damage to persons or property arising out of or related to any use of the material contained in this book.

The Publisher

Library of Congress Cataloging-in-Publication Data

Ferri, Fred F.
  Ferri's best test : a practical guide to clinical laboratory medicine and diagnostic imaging / Fred F. Ferri. — 2nd ed.
    p. ; cm.
  Includes bibliographical references and index.
  ISBN 978-0-323-05759-2
  1. Diagnosis, Laboratory—Handbooks, manuals, etc. 2. Diagnostic imaging—Handbooks, manuals, etc. I. Title. II. Title: Best test. III.
Title: Practical guide to clinical laboratory medicine and diagnostic imaging.
  [DNLM: 1. Clinical Laboratory Techniques—Handbooks. 2. Diagnostic Imaging—Handbooks. 3. Reference Values—Handbooks. QY 39 F388f 2010]
  RB38.2.F47 2010
  616.07'5—dc22

2008040453

Acquisitions Editor: James Merritt
Developmental Editor: Nicole DiCicco
Project Manager: Bryan Hayward
Design Direction: Gene Harris

Printed in China

Working together to grow
libraries in developing countries
www.elsevier.com | www.bookaid.org | www.sabre.org

ELSEVIER   BOOK AID International   Sabre Foundation

Last digit is the print number: 9 8 7 6 5 4 3 2 1

ACKNOWLEDGMENTS

I extend a special thank you to the authors and contributors of the following texts who have lent multiple images, illustrations, and text material to this book:

Grainger RG, Allison D: *Grainger & Allison's Diagnostic Radiology, a Textbook of Medical Imaging*, ed 4, Philadelphia: Churchill Livingstone, 2001
Mettler FA: *Primary Care Radiology*, Philadelphia, WB Saunders, 2000
Pagana KD, Pagana TJ: *Mosby's Diagnostic and Laboratory Test Reference*, ed 8, St. Louis, Mosby, 2007
Talley NJ, Martin CJ: *Clinical Gastroenterology*, ed 2, Sidney, Churchill Livingstone, 2006
Weissleder R, Wittenberg J, Harisinghani MG, Chen JW: *Primer of Diagnostic Imaging*, ed 4, St. Louis, Mosby, 2007
Wu AHB: *Tietz Clinical Guide to Laboratory Tests*, Philadelphia, WB Saunders, 2006

Fred F. Ferri, MD, FACP
Clinical Professor
Alpert Medical School
Brown University
Providence, Rhode Island

PREFACE

This book is intended to be a practical and concise guide to clinical laboratory medicine and diagnostic imaging. It is designed for use by medical students, interns, residents, practicing physicians, and other health care personnel who deal with laboratory testing and diagnostic imaging in their daily work.

As technology evolves, physicians are faced with a constantly changing armamentarium of diagnostic imaging and laboratory tests to supplement their clinical skills in arriving at a correct diagnosis. In addition, with the advent of managed care it is increasingly important for physicians to practice cost-effective medicine.

The aim of this book is to be a practical reference for ordering tests, whether they are laboratory tests or diagnostic imaging studies. As such it is unique in medical publishing. This manual is divided into three main sections: clinical laboratory testing, diagnostic imaging, and diagnostic algorithms.

Section I deals with common diagnostic imaging tests. Each test is approached with the following format: Indications, Strengths, Weaknesses, and Comments. The approximate cost of each test is also indicated. For the second edition, we have added several new additional diagnostic modalities such as computed tomographic colonography (virtual colonoscopy), CT/PET scan, and video capsule endoscopy.

Section II has been greatly expanded with the addition of 113 tests, for a total of 313 laboratory tests. Each test is approached with the following format:
- Laboratory test
- Normal range in adult patients
- Common abnormalities (e.g., positive test, increased or decreased value)
- Causes of abnormal result

Section III includes the diagnostic modalities (imaging and laboratory tests) and algorithms of common diseases and disorders. This section has been expanded with the addition of 9 new algorithms for a total of 231.

I hope that this unique approach will simplify the diagnostic testing labyrinth and will lead the readers of this manual to choose the best test to complement their clinical skills. However, it is important to remember that lab tests and x-rays do not make diagnoses, doctors do. As such, any lab and radiographic results should be integrated with the complete clinical picture to arrive at a diagnosis.

Fred F. Ferri, MD, FACP

CONTENTS

SECTION II   Laboratory values and interpretation of results

xii Contents

Contents xv

Contents xix

Section III Diseases and disorders

Diagnostic Imaging

This section deals with common diagnostic imaging tests. Each test is approached with the following format: Indications, Strengths, Weaknesses, Comments. The comparative cost of each test is also indicated. Please note that there is considerable variation in the charges and reimbursement for each diagnostic imaging procedure based on individual insurance and geographic region. The cost described in this book is based on RBRVS fee schedule provided by the Center for Medicare & Medicaid Services for total component billing.

$ Relatively inexpensive $$$$$Very expensive

1. Abdominal Film, Plain (Kidney, Ureter, and Bladder [KUB])

Indications
- Abdominal pain
- Suspected intraperitoneal free air (pneumoperitoneum) (Fig. 1-1)
- Bowel distention

Strengths
- Low cost
- Readily available
- Low radiation

Weaknesses
- Low diagnostic yield
- Contraindicated in pregnancy
- Presence of barium from recent radiographs will interfere with interpretation
- Nonspecific test

Comments
- KUB is a coned plain radiograph of the abdomen, which includes kidneys, ureters, and bladder.
- A typical abdominal series includes flat and upright radiographs.
- KUB is valuable as a preliminary study when investigating abdominal pain/pathology (e.g., pneumoperitoneum, bowel obstruction, calcifications). Fig. 1-2 describes a normal gas pattern
- This is the least expensive but also least sensitive method to assess bowel obstruction radiographically.
- Cost: $

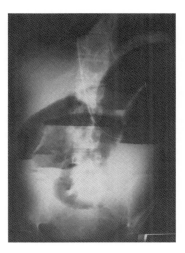

Figure 1-1 Plain abdominal x-ray examination of small bowel obstruction showing distended loops of small bowel with multiple fluid levels and absence of colonic gas. *(From NJ Talley, CJ Martin: Clinical Gastroenterology, ed 2, Sidney, Churchill Livingstone, 2006.)*

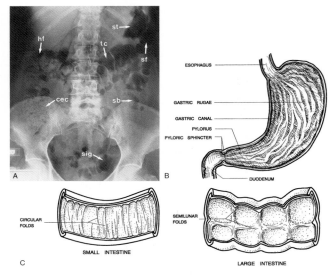

Figure 1-2 **A** to **C**, Normal bowel gas pattern. Gas is normally swallowed and can be seen in the stomach *(st)*. Small amounts of air normally can be seen in the small bowel *(sb)*, usually in the left midabdomen or the central portion of the abdomen. In this patient, gas can be seen throughout the entire colon, including the cecum *(cec)*. In the area where the air is mixed with feces, there is a mottled pattern. Cloverleaf-shaped collections of air are seen in the hepatic flexure *(hf)*, transverse colon *(tc)*, splenic flexure *(sf)*, and sigmoid *(sig)*. *(From Mettler FA: Primary Care Radiology, Philadelphia, WB Saunders, 2000.)*

2. Barium Enema

Indications
- Colorectal carcinoma
- Diverticular disease (Fig. 1-3)
- Inflammatory bowel disease
- Lower GI bleeding
- Polyposis syndromes
- Constipation
- Evaluation of for leak of postsurgical anastomotic site

Strengths
- Readily available
- Inexpensive
- Good visualization of mucosal detail with double-contrast barium enema (DCBE)

Weaknesses
- Uncomfortable bowel preparation and procedure for most patients
- Risk of bowel perforation
- Contraindicated in pregnancy
- Can result in severe postprocedure constipation in elderly patients
- Poorly cleansed bowel will interfere with interpretation
- Poor visualization of rectosigmoid lesions

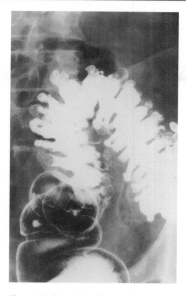

Figure 1-3 Diverticular disease showing typical muscle changes in the sigmoid and diverticula arising from the apices of the clefts between interdigitating muscle folds. *(From Grainger RG, Allison D: Grainger & Allison's Diagnostic Radiology: A Textbook of Medical Imaging, Churchill Livingstone, ed 4, 2001.)*

Comments

- Barium enema is now rarely performed or indicated. Colonoscopy is more sensitive and specific for evaluation of suspected colorectal lesions.
- This test should not be performed in patients with suspected free perforation, fulminant colitis, severe pseudomembranous colitis, or toxic megacolon or in a setting of acute diverticulitis.
- A single-contrast BE uses thin barium to fill the colon, whereas DCBE uses thick barium to coat the colon and air to distend the lumen. Single-contrast BE is generally used to rule out diverticulosis, whereas DCBE is preferable for evaluating colonic mucosa, detecting small lesions, and diagnosing inflammatory bowel disease.
- Cost: $$

3. Barium Swallow (Esophagram)

Indications

- Achalasia
- Esophageal neoplasm (primary or metastatic)
- Esophageal diverticuli (e.g., Zenker diverticulum), pseudodiverticuli
- Suspected aspiration, evaluation for aspiration following stroke
- Suspected anastomotic leak

- Esophageal stenosis/obstruction
- Extrinsic esophageal compression
- Dysphagia
- Esophageal tear/perforation
- Fistula (aortoesophageal, tracheoesophageal)
- Esophagitis (infectious, chemical)
- Mucosal ring (e.g., Schatzki ring)
- Esophageal webs (e.g., Plummer-Vinson syndrome)

Strengths
- Low cost
- Readily available

Weaknesses
- Contraindicated in pregnancy
- Requires patient cooperation
- Radiation exposure

Comments
- In a barium swallow study, the radiologist observes the swallowing mechanism while films of the cervical and thoracic esophagus are obtained.

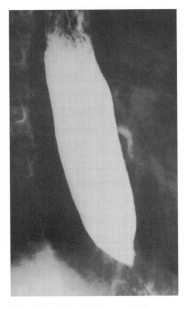

Figure 1-4 Radiograph of oesophageal achalasia showing the typical tapered ('bird beaked') appearance at the cardio-oesophageal junction and retention of food and fluid within a dilated and adynamic oesophagus. *(From Talley NJ, Martin CJ: Clinical Gastroenterology, ed 2, Sidney, Churchill Livingstone, 2006.)*

- Barium is generally used because it provides better anatomic detail than water-soluble contrast agents; however, diatrizoate (Hypaque) or gastrograffin should be used rather than barium sulfate in suspected perforation or anastomotic leak because free barium in the peritoneal cavity induces a granulomatous response that can result in adhesions/peritonitis or in the mediastinum can result in mediastinitis.
- Cost: $

4. Upper GI Series (UGI)

Indications
- Gastroesophageal reflux disease (GERD)
- Peptic ulcer disease
- Esophageal carcinoma
- Gastric carcinoma (Fig. 1-5)
- Gastric lymphoma
- Gastric polyps
- Gastritis (hypertrophic, erosive, infectious, granulomatous)
- Gastric outlet obstruction
- Gastroparesis
- Metastatic neoplasm (from colon, liver, pancreas, melanoma)
- Congenital abnormalities (e.g., hypertrophic pyloric stenosis, antral mucosal diaphragm)
- Evaluation for complications after gastric surgery

Strengths
- Inexpensive
- Readily available

Weaknesses
- Contraindicated in pregnancy
- Can result in significant post-procedure constipation in elderly patients
- Requires patient cooperation
- Radiation exposure

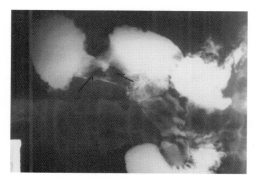

Figure 1-5 Gastric adenocarcinoma of the stomach. (*From Talley NJ, Martin CJ: Clinical Gastroenterology, ed 2, Sidney, Churchill Livingstone, 2006.*)

Comments

- Upper endoscopy is invasive and more expensive but is more sensitive and has replaced UGI series for evaluation of esophageal and gastric lesions.
- In a barium swallow examination, only films of the cervical and thoracic esophagus are obtained, whereas in an UGI series films are taken of the thoracic esophagus, stomach, and duodenal bulb.
- Barium provides better anatomic detail than water-soluble contrast agents; however, water-soluble contrast agents (Gastrografin, Hypaque) are preferred when perforation is suspected or postoperatively to assess anastomosis for leaks or obstruction because free barium in the peritoneal cavity can produce a granulomatous response that can result in adhesions.
- It is necessary to clean out the stomach with nasogastric (NG) suction before performing contrast examination when gastric outlet obstruction is suspected.
- Cost: $$

5. Computed Tomographic Colonoscopy (CTC, Virtual Colonoscopy)

Indications
- Screening for colorectal carcinoma

Strengths
- May be more acceptable to patients than fiber-optic colonoscopy
- Does not require sedation
- Safer than fiber-optic colonoscopy
- Lower cost than fiber-optic colonoscopy
- Standard examination does not require intravenous (IV) contrast
- Also visualizes abdomen and lower thorax and can detect abnormalities there (e.g., aortic aneurysms, cancers of ovary, pancreas, lung, liver, kidney)

Weaknesses
- Failure to detect clinically important flat lesions, which do not protrude into the lumen of the colon
- Need for cathartic preparation; requires the same bowel preparation as colonoscopy
- Lack of therapeutic ability; nearly 10% of patients will require follow-up traditional colonoscopies due to abnormalities detected by CTC
- Most insurance companies will not pay for procedure
- Incidental findings detected on CTC can lead to additional and often unnecessary testing
- Radiation Exposure

Comments
- CTC uses a CT scanner to take a series of radiographs of the colon and a computer to create a three-dimensional (3-D) view. It can be uncomfortable because the patient isn't sedated and a small tube is inserted in the rectum to inflate the colon so that it can be more easily viewed
- CTC uses a low-dose x-ray technique, typically 20% of the radiation used with standard diagnostic CT, and approximately 10% less than double-competent barium enema.
- Most insurance companies do not pay for CTC, but that could change if colon cancer screening guidelines endorse it.
- Sensitivity ranges from 85% to 94% and specificity is approximately 96% for detecting large ($\geq$ 1 cm) polyps.
- Cost: $$$

6. CT of Abdomen/Pelvis

Indications
- Evaluation of abdominal mass, pelvic mass
- Suspected lymphoma
- Staging of neoplasm of abdominal/pelvic organs
- Splenomegaly
- Intraabdominal, pelvic, or retroperitoneal abscess (Fig. 1-6)
- Abdominal/pelvic trauma
- Jaundice
- Pancreatitis
- Suspected bowel obstruction
- Appendicitis

Strengths
- Fast
- Noninvasive

Weaknesses
- Potential for significant contrast reaction
- Suboptimal sensitivity for traumatic injury of the pancreas, diaphragm, small bowel, and mesentery
- Retained barium from other studies will interfere with interpretation
- Expensive
- Relatively contraindicated in pregnancy
- Radiation exposure

Comments
- CT with contrast is the initial diagnostic imaging of choice in patients with left lower quadrant (LLQ) and right lower quadrant (RLQ) abdominal pain/mass in adults. Ultrasound is preferred as initial imaging modality in children, young

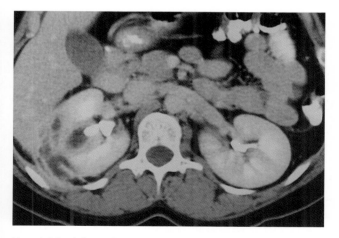

Figure 1-6 Renal abscess. Contrast computed tomography shows an abscess in the medulla of the kidney with penetration and extension into the perinephric space *(arrows)*. *(From Johnson RJ, Feehally J: Comprehensive Clinical Nephrology, ed 2, St. Louis, Mosby, 2000.)*

women, and in evaluation of right upper quadrant (RUQ) and mid-abdominal pain/mass unless the patient is significantly obese
- CT of abdomen/pelvis with contrast is the imaging procedure of choice for suspected abdominal abscess in adults.
- CT is 90% sensitive for small bowel obstruction.
- Fig. 1-7 describes various images seen on CT of abdomen. The orientation of CT and magnetic resonance (MR) images is described in Fig. 1-8.
- Cost: CT without contrast $$; CT with contrast $$$; CT with and without contrast $$$

7. Helical or Spiral CT of Abdomen/Pelvis

Indications
- Suspected acute appendicitis
- Abdominal/pelvic pain
- Abdominal/pelvic neoplasm (primary or metastatic)
- Abdominal/pelvic mass
- Abdominal/pelvic abscess
- Suspected complication from acute pancreatitis (e.g., abscess, pseudocyst)

Strengths
- Fast (reduced scan time—important for critically ill patients)
- Imaging of entire abdomen and pelvis in a single breath hold
- Better imaging than conventional CT
- Not affected by overlying gas (unlike ultrasound)

Weaknesses
- Potential for significant contrast reaction
- Expensive
- Lacks sensitivity in diagnosis and staging of urologic cancers in the pelvis
- Radiation exposure

Comments
- CT is an excellent modality for diagnosing calculi in kidneys and ureters without IV contrast.
- CT is useful for evaluation of renal masses and retroperitoneal lesion.
- Cost: CT of abdomen without contrast $$; CT of abdomen with contrast $$$; CT of pelvis with contrast $$$

8. Hepatobiliary (Iminodiacetic Acid [IDA]) Scan

Indications
- Acute cholecystitis
- Chronic acalculous cholecystitis
- Bile leak
- Postcholecystectomy syndrome
- Obstruction of bile flow
- Biliary dyskinesia
- Biliary atresia
- Afferent loop syndrome
- Evaluation of focal liver lesions

Strengths
- Not operator dependent
- High specificity for excluding acute cholecystitis

Weaknesses
- Severe hepatocellular dysfunction with bilirubin greater than 20 mg/dl will result in poor excretion and nondiagnostic study

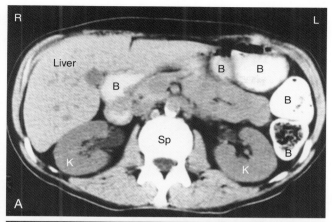

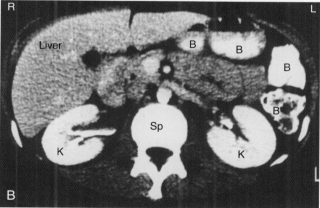

Figure 1-7 Computed tomography. Images of the abdomen are presented here. **A,** The image is done with the use of relatively wide windows during filming, and no intravenous contrast material is used. **B,** The windows are narrowed, producing a rather grainy image, and intravenous contrast material is administered so that you can see enhancement of the aorta, abdominal vessels, and both kidneys *(K)*. In both images, contrast material is used in the bowel *(B)* to differentiate the bowel from solid organs and structures. *Sp,* spine. *(From Mettler FA: Primary Care Radiology. Philadelphia, WB Saunders, 2000.)*

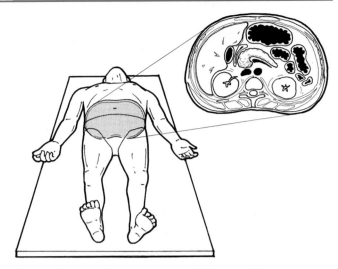

Figure 1-8 Orientation of computed tomography (CT) and magnetic resonance (MR) images. CT and MR usually present images as transverse (axial) slices of the body. The orientation of most slices is the same as that of a patient viewed from the foot of the bed. *(From Mettler FA: Primary Care Radiology. Philadelphia, WB Saunders, 2000.)*

- Recent or concomitant use of opiates or meperidine may interfere with bile flow
- False positives common
- Time consuming (requires more than 1 hour of actual imaging time and patient preparation)

Comments
- In a normal scan, the radiopharmaceutical is cleared from the blood pool after 5 minutes, there is noticeable liver clearing after 30 minutes, and gallbladder and bowel activity is visualized after 60 minutes. Images are obtained every 5 minutes for 1 hour. Late images can be obtained for up to 4 hours after injection. Nonvisualization of the gallbladder is indicative of cholecystitis (Fig. 1-9).
- •This test is most helpful when clinical suspicion for cholecystitis is high and ultrasound results are inconclusive.
- Food intake will interfere with test. Optimal fasting is 4 to 12 hours. Fasting longer than 24 hours will also lead to inconclusive exam.
- Cost: $$$

9. Endoscopic Retrograde Cholangiopancreatography (ERCP)

Indications
- Evaluation and treatment of diseases of the bile ducts and pancreas
- Treatment of choice for bile duct stones (Fig. 1-10) and for immediate relief of extrahepatic biliary obstruction in benign disease

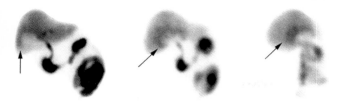

Figure 1-9 Acute cholecystitis, hot rim sign *(arrows)*, is suspicious for gangrenous gallbladder. Curvilinear area of relatively increased activity in liver adjacent to gallbladder *(GB)* persists in delayed images. Anterior, right anterior oblique, and right lateral views start at 40 minutes after injection. GB did not visualize at 4 hours (not shown). *(From Specht N: Practical guide to diagnostic imaging, St. Louis, Mosby, 1998.)*

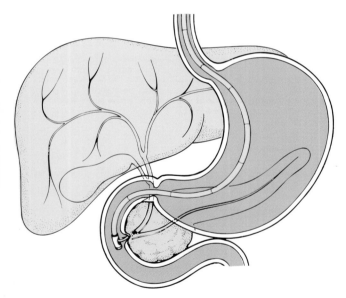

Figure 1-10 Endoscopic retrograde cholangiopancreatography. The fiberoptic scope is passed into the duodenum. Note the small catheter being advances into the biliary duct. *(From Pagana KD, Pagana, TJ: Mosby's Diagnostic and Laboratory Test Reference, ed 8, St. Louis, Mosby, 2007.)*

- Other indications are biliary obstruction due to cancer, acute and recurrent pancreatitis, pancreatic pseudocyst, suspected sphincter of Oddi dysfunction
- Can be used for diagnostic purposes when MRCP and other imaging studies are inconclusive or unreliable, such as in suspected cases of primary sclerosing cholangitis early in the disease, when the changes in duct morphology are

subtle, or in patient with nondilated bile duct and clinical signs and symptoms highly suggestive of gallstone or biliary sludge
- Preferred modality in patients with high pretest probability of sphincter dysfunction or ampullary stenosis

Strengths
- Preferred modality for treatment of bile duct stones (Fig. 1-11)
- Well suited to evaluate for and treat bile duct leaks and biliary tract injury after open or laparoscopic biliary surgery
- ERCP in management of pancreatic and biliary cancer allows access to obstructed bile and pancreatic ducts for collecting tissue samples and placement of stents to temporarily relieve obstruction

Weaknesses
- Invasive, technically difficult procedure
- 5% to 7% risk of pancreatitis depending on patient, procedure, and operator expertise. Other complications, such as bleeding, cholangitis, cholecystitis, cardiopulmonary events, perforation, and death occur far less often

Comments
- In ERCP, contrast-agent injection is performed through the endoscope after cannulation of the common bile duct. Complications include pancreatitis, duodenal perforation, and GI bleeding.
- Although the complication rate of ERCP is acceptable when compared with other invasive procedures such as biliary bypass surgery or open bile duct exploration, the rate is too high for patients with a low pretest probability of disease if the procedure is to be done purely diagnostically.
- Centers that perform a significant volume of ERCP have higher completion rates and lower complication rates.
- Cost: $$$$

10. Percutaneous Biliary Procedures

Indications
- Transhepatic cholangiogram: used for demonstration of biliary anatomy, first step before biliary drainage or stent placement

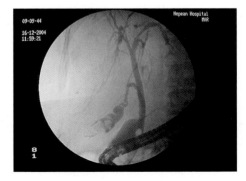

Figure 1-11 Endoscopic retrograde cholangiopancreatography demonstrating gallstones within the gallbladder and common bile duct. *(From Talley NJ, Martin CJ: Clinical Gastroenterology, ed 2, Sidney, Churchill Livingstone, 2006.)*

- Biliary drainage: used for biliary obstruction
- Biliary stent placement: used for malignant biliary stricture (Fig. 1-12), inability to place endoscopic stent

Weaknesses
- Invasive
- Operator dependent
- Cost: $$$$

11. Magnetic Resonance Cholangiography (MRCP)

Indications
- Suspected biliary or pancreatic disease
- Unsuccessful ERCP, contraindication to ERCP, and presence of biliary enteric anastomoses (e.g., choledocojejunostomy, Billroth II anastomosis)

Strengths
- Advantages over ERCP: noninvasive, less expensive, requires no radiation, less operator dependent, allows better visualization of ducts proximal to obstruction,

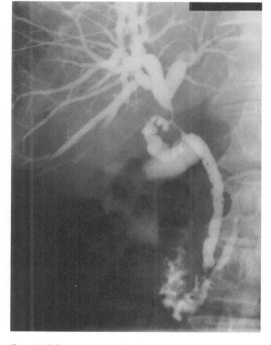

Figure 1-12 Percutaneous transhepatic cholangiography (PTC) in hilar tumor assessment. Relatively undistended ducts in a patient with a cholangiocarcinoma; a short stricture involves the junction of the common hepatic and common bile ducts. *(From Grainger RG, Allison D: Grainger & Allison's Diagnostic Radiology: A Textbook of Medical Imaging, Churchill Livingstone, ed 4, 2001.)*

and can allow detection of extraductal disease when combined with conventional T1W and T2W sequences
- Useful in patients who have biliary or pancreatic pain but no objective abnormalities in liver tests or routine imaging studies
- Can detect retained stone with sensitivity of 92% and specificity of 97%

Weaknesses
- Limitations of MRCP include artifacts due to surgical clips, pneumobilia, or duodenal diverticuli, and use in patients with implantable devices or claustrophobia
- Accuracy diminished by stones 1 mm or less and normal bile duct diameter (< 8 mm)
- Decreased spatial resolution makes MRCP less sensitive to abnormalities of the peripheral intrahepatic ducts (e.g., sclerosing cholangitis) and pancreatic ductal side branches (e.g., chronic pancreatitis)
- Cannot perform therapeutic endoscopic or percutaneous interventions for obstructing bile duct lesions; thus, in patients with high clinical suspicion for bile duct obstruction, ERCP should be initial imaging modality to provide timely intervention (e.g., sphincterectomy, dilatation, stent placement, stone removal) if necessary
- Pitfalls include pseudofilling defects, pseudodilations, and nonvisualization of ducts

Comments
- Overall sensitivity of MRCP for biliary obstruction is 95%. The procedure is less sensitive for stones (92%) and malignant conditions (92%) than for the presence of obstruction.
- Cost: $$$$

12. Meckel Scan (TC-99m Pertechnetate Scintigraphy)

Indication
- Identification of Meckel's diverticulum

Strengths
- In children, overall sensitivity for Meckel's diverticulum is 85%; specificity is 95%; sensitivity lower in adults (63%)

Weaknesses
- False negative studies may occur due to lack of sufficient gastric mucosa, poor technique, or washout of secreted pertechnetate
- False positives can be due to several factors, including atrioventricular (AV) malformations, peptic ulcer, inflammatory bowel disease (IBD), neoplasms, and hydronephrosis
- Barium in GI tract from prior studies may mask radionuclide concentration

Comments
- Meckel's diverticulum appears scintigraphically as a focal area of increased intraperitoneal activity usually 5 to 10 minutes after tracer injection.
- Full stomach or urinary bladder may obscure an adjacent Meckel's diverticulum; therefore fasting for 4 hours and voiding before, during, and after scan are important.
- Cost: $$

13. MRI of Abdomen

Indications
- Suspected liver hemangioma
- Evaluation of adrenal mass

- Cervical cancer staging
- Endometrial cancer staging (Fig. 1-13)
- Evaluation of renal mass in patients allergic to iodine and in patients with diminished renal function
- Staging of renal cell carcinoma
- Evaluation of Müllerian duct anomalies when ultrasound is equivocal
- Characterization of pelvic mass indeterminate on ultrasound
- Evaluation of hepatic mass

Strengths
- Noninvasive
- Generally safe contrast agent (MRI uses gadolinium, an IV agent that is less nephrotoxic)
- No ionizing radiation

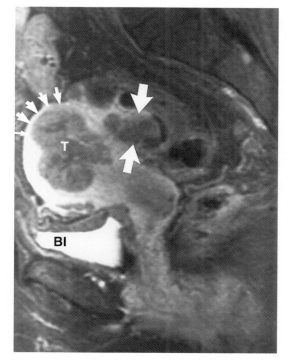

Figure 1-13 Endometrial carcinoma. The sagittal gadolinium-enhanced T1-weighted fat-suppressed spoiled GRE MR image, shows an endometrial cancer *(T)* with deep myometrial invasion. Note the thin rim of normal myometrium *(small arrows)*. The disease extends to the adnexae *(large arrows)* (B1, bladder). (From Grainger RG, Allison D: Grainger & Allison's Diagnostic Radiology: a Textbook of Medical Imaging, Churchill Livingstone, ed 4, 2001.)

- Soft tissue resolution
- Multiplanar

Weaknesses
- Expensive
- Needs cooperative patient
- Time consuming
- Cannot be performed in patients with non–MR-compatible aneurysm clips, pacemaker, cochlear implants, or metallic foreign body in eyes; safe in women with intrauterine devices (IUDs), including copper ones, and those with surgical clips and staples

Comments
- In patients with chronic liver disease, MRI is more sensitive (81% sensitivity) but less specific (85% specificity) than ultrasonography (sensitivity 61%, specificity 97%) or spiral CT (sensitivity 68%, specificity 93%) for diagnosis of hepatocellular carcinoma.
- Anxious patients (especially those with claustrophobia) should be premedicated with an anxiolitic agent, and imaging should be done with "open MRI" whenever possible.
- Cost: MRI with and without contrast $$$$$

14. Small-Bowel Series

Indications
- Small-bowel lymphoma and other small-bowel neoplasms
- Malabsorption
- Inflammatory bowel disease
- Celiac sprue
- "Short-bowel" syndrome
- Pancreatic insufficiency
- Intestinal fistula
- GI bleeding
- Anemia (if other tests are negative or non-contributory)

Strengths
- Inexpensive
- Readily available
- Good visualization of mucosal detail

Weaknesses
- Contraindicated in pregnancy
- Requires cooperative patient
- Time consuming
- Radiation exposure

Comments
- In a small-bowel series, sequential films are obtained at 15- to 30-minute intervals until the terminal ileum is visualized with fluoroscopy and spot films.
- Cost: $$

15. TC-99m Sulfur Colloid Scintigraphy (TC-99m sc) for GI Bleeding

Indications
- Localization of GI bleeding of undetermined source

Strengths
- Fast: in patient who is actively bleeding, this 20-minute study can be promptly performed and completed before angiography
- Active hemorrhage is most commonly detected in first 5 to 10 minutes of imaging

- In addition to detecting bleeding site, may also detect other abnormalities such as vascular blushes of tumors, angiodysplasia, and arteriovenous malformations

Weaknesses
- Main disadvantage is that bleeding must be active (bleeding rate > 0.1 ml/min) at time of injection
- Inexact localization of bleeding site. Because blood acts as an intestinal irritant, movement can often be rapid and bi-directional, making it difficult to localize site of bleeding
- Ectopic spleen and asymmetric bone marrow activity can interfere with detection of bleeding
- Presence of barium in GI tract may obscure bleeding site

Comments
- After injection of Tc-99m SC, radiotracer will extravasate at the bleeding site into the lumen with each recirculation of blood. The site of bleeding is seen as a focal area of radiotracer accumulation that increases in intensity and moves through the GI tract.
- Tc-99mSC is less sensitive than Tc-99 red blood cell scan and is used less often for evaluation of GI hemorrhage.
- Cost: $$

16. TC-99m–Labeled Red Blood Cell (RBC) Scintigraphy for GI Bleeding

Indications
- Localization of GI bleeding of undetermined source

Strengths
- Major advantage over Tc-99m SC is that a hemorrhagic site can be detected over much longer period and can reimage if bleeding not seen immediately and patient rebleeds
- In addition to detecting active bleeding sites, may be able to detect vascular blushes of tumors, angiodysplasia and AV malformations

Weaknesses
- False positive results due to misinterpretation of normal variants or poorly detailed delayed images
- Time-consuming; not indicated in patient actively bleeding and clinically unstable
- Inexact localization of bleeding site; because blood acts as an intestinal irritant, movement can often be rapid and bi-directional, making it difficult to localize site of bleeding
- Presence of barium in GI tract may obscure bleeding site
- Visualization requires a bleeding rate greater than 0.1 ml/min

Comments
- In an RBC scan, the patient's RBCs are collected, labeled with a radioisotope, and then returned to the patient's circulation.
- Criteria for positive Tc-RBC scintigraphy are as follows: abnormal radiotracer "hot" spot appears and conforms to bowel anatomy, there is persistence or increase in normal activity over time (Fig. 1-14), and there is noticeable movement of activity by peristalsis, retrograde, or anterograde.
- Cost: $$

17. Ultrasound of Abdomen

Indications
- Abdominal pain
- Jaundice

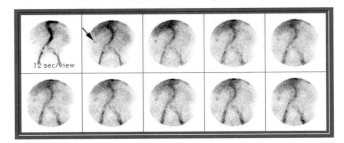

Figure 1-14 Acute GI bleed, Tc-99m RBC. Anterior dynamic images show tortuous arteriosclerotic aorta and common iliac arteries, with early, persistent focus of activity in right upper quadrant of abdomen *(arrow)*. *(From Specht N: Practical Guide to Diagnostic Imaging, St. Louis, Mosby, 1998.)*

- Cholelithiasis (Fig. 1-15)
- Cholecystitis
- Elevated liver enzymes
- Splenomegaly
- Ascites
- Abdominal mass

Strengths
- Fast
- Can be performed at bedside (Fig. 1-16)
- No ionizing radiation
- Widely available
- Can provide Doppler and color flow information
- Lower cost than CT

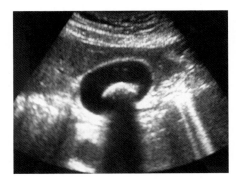

Figure 1-15 Ultrasound demonstrating a single large gallstone within the gallbladder. Note the typical shadowing below the stone. *(From Talley NJ, Martin CJ: Clinical Gastroenterology, ed 2, Sidney, Churchill Livingstone, 2006.)*

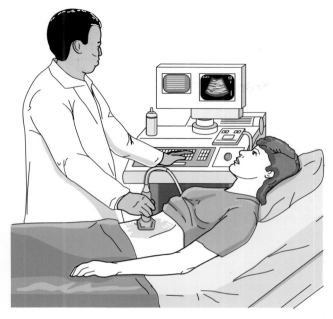

Figure 1-16 Ultrasound of the abdomen. *(From Pagana KD, Pagana, TJ: Mosby's Diagnostic and Laboratory Test Reference, ed 8, St. Louis, Mosby, 2007.)*

Weaknesses
- Obscuring intestinal gas
- Inferior anatomic detail compared with CT
- Affected by body habitus
- Cannot be used to definitely rule out abscess

Comments
- This is often the initial diagnostic procedure of choice in patients presenting with abdominal pain or mass in RUQ and mid-abdomen. CT of abdomen is preferred in LLQ and RLQ pain or mass and in significantly obese patients.
- Cost: $$

18. Ultrasound of Appendix

Indications
- Suspected appendicitis

Strengths
- Fast
- Readily available
- Noninvasive
- No ionizing radiation

Weaknesses
- Can be affected by overlying bowel gas and body habitus (e.g., obese patient)
- Operator dependent; results may be affected by skill of technician

Comments
- This is the best initial study in suspected appendicitis in children and pregnant patients.
- Cost: $$

19. Ultrasound of Gallbladder and Bile Ducts

Indications
- Suspected cholelithiasis
- Cholecystitis
- Gallbladder polyps
- Gallbladder neoplasms
- Choledocholithiasis
- Biliary neoplasm
- Cholangitis
- Suspected congenital biliary abnormalities (e.g., biliary atresia, Caroli's disease, choledochal cyst)
- Biliary dyskinesia

Strengths
- Fast
- Readily available
- Can be performed at bedside
- Noninvasive
- No ionizing radiation

Weaknesses
- Is affected by overlying bowel gas and body habitus (e.g., obese patient)
- Operator dependent; results may be affected by skill of technician

Comments
- This is the initial best test for suspected cholelithiasis and cholecystitis.
- Patient must take nothing by mouth for 4 hours but not greater than 24 hours (gallbladder may be contracted).
- Cost: $$

20. Ultrasound of Liver

Indications
- Elevated liver enzymes
- Hepatomegaly
- Liver mass (neoplasm, cystic disease, abscess)
- Jaundice
- Hepatic trauma
- Hepatic hemangioma
- Hepatic parenchymal disease (e.g., fatty infiltration, hemochromatosis, hepatitis, cirrhosis, portal hypertension)
- Ascites

Strengths
- Fast
- Widely available
- Portable (can be performed at bedside)
- Noninvasive
- No ionizing radiation
- Low cost

Weaknesses
- Can be affected by overlying bowel gas and body habitus
- Cannot be used to definitely rule out abscess
- Rib artifact may obscure images of the right lobe
- Rarely provides definitive diagnosis and usually requires confirmatory CT or MRI

Comments
- Due to its widespread availability, noninvasive nature, and low cost, ultrasound is often performed as initial study in evaluation of suspected liver disease.
- Cost: $$

21. Ultrasound of Pancreas

Indications
- Pancreatitis
- Cystic fibrosis
- Pancreatic abscess
- Pancreatic pseudocyst
- Suspected neoplasm
- Trauma

Strengths
- Fast
- Noninvasive
- Can be performed at bedside
- No ionizing radiation

Weaknesses
- Is affected by overlying bowel gas and body habitus (e.g., in obese patient fat overlying the pancreas impedes visualization)
- Operator dependent; results may be affected by skill of technician
- Barium from recent radiographs will interfere with visualization
- Cannot be used to conclusively rule out abscess
- Difficult to evaluate tail of pancreas due to location

Comments
- Cost: $$

22. Endoscopic Ultrasound (EUS)

Indications
- Evaluation of choledocholithiasis
- Pre-operative staging of esophageal malignancies
- Detection of defects in internal and external sphincter in patients with fecal incontinence, detection of exophytic distal rectal tumors, fistula-in-ano, peri-anal abscess, rectal ulcer, and presacral cyst
- Localization of insulinomas and other pancreatic endocrine tumors
- Evaluation of submucosal lesions of the GI tract
- Guidance for fine needle aspiration of pancreatic cysts
- Chronic pancreatitis: useful to delineate strictures and proximal dilatation of CBD and intrahepatic biliary radicles

Strengths
- When used for evaluation of submucosal GI lesions, the sensitivity of EUS in determining the depth of tumor invasion is about 85% to 90%
- In fecal incontinence, EUS –detected sphincter disruption correlates well with pressure measurements and operative findings
- EUS is less invasive than MRCP and has a sensitivity and specificity of 90% to 100% for evaluation of choledocholithiasis

Weaknesses
- Can overestimate the extent of GI tumor invasion due to the presence of tissue inflammation and edema
- Operator dependent, results may be affected by skill of technician

Comments
- EUS involves visualization of the GI tract via a high frequency ultrasound transducer placed through an endoscope
- Cost: $$$

23. Video Capsule Endoscopy (VCE)

Indications
- Determination of obscure source of GI bleeding
- Diagnosis of Crohn's disease in the small intestine
- Detection of tumors and polyps in the small bowel
- Diagnosis of Meckel's diverticulum
- Diagnosis of small-bowel varices in patients with portal hypertension and obscure GI bleeding

Strengths
- Noninvasive
- Ambulatory testing
- Minimal or no patient discomfort
- Able to visualize the entire small intestine
- Does not require sedation or analgesia

Weaknesses
- Cannot take biopsies
- Can result in capsule retention (<1%) requiring surgical intervention if there is an obstruction or stricture
- Labor intensive for endoscopist (50-100 minutes to review images)
- Relatively contraindicated in patients with implanted pacemakers or defibrillators (possible interference)

Comments
- In VCE, the patient fasts for 12 hours then swallows a miniature high-resolution camera that is propelled through the GI tract, allowing visualization of the small intestine inaccessible by conventional endoscopy. The capsule measures 11×23 mm and contains a color video camera and transmitters. The patient wears sensors and a data recorder. The capsule is propelled by peristalsis through the GI tract and acquires two or more video images per second. The capsule is used once and is not recovered. When the study is completed, the stored images are downloaded to a computer for viewing.
- Diagnostic yield for obscure GI bleeding is 50% to 70%.
- Cost: $$$

B.   Breast Imaging

1. Mammogram

Indications
- Screening for breast cancer. American Cancer Society guidelines recommend:
  Baseline mammogram, age 35 to 40
  Yearly mammogram after age 40
  Under age 30, mammography generally not indicated unless positive family history of breast cancer at a very early age
- Evaluation of breast mass, tenderness

Strengths
- Inexpensive
- Readily available

Weaknesses
- Misses 15% to 20% of breast neoplasms
- Can be painful for patient
- Poor identification of nonpalpable intraductal papillomas
- Residue on breasts from powders, deodorants, or perfumes may interfere with diagnosis of lesions

Comments
- Digital mammography is the single best initial method for detecting breast cancer (Fig. 1-17) in a curable stage based on cost and availability.
- When ordering a mammogram, it is important to distinguish a screening mammogram from a diagnostic mammogram. Screening mammograms are indicated in healthy women (see guidelines earlier), whereas a diagnostic mammogram is indicated when patients present with signs or symptoms related to the breast or palpable abnormalities on breast examination.
- Mammography is available in both plain film and digital format. Digital mammography is often performed because it offers the following advantages over film mammography: significantly shorter exam times, 50% less radiation than traditional film radiography, 27% more sensitive for cancer in women under 50 and in women with dense breast tissue.
- The use of computer-aided detection in screening mammography is associated with reduced accuracy of interpretation of screening mammograms. The increased rate of biopsy with the use of computer-aided detection is not clearly associated with improved detection of invasive breast cancer.
- Cost: $

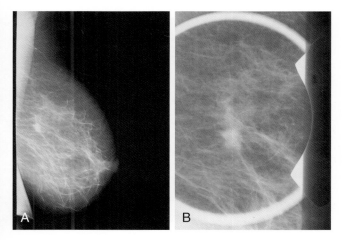

Figure 1-17 Right mediolateral (**A**) and spot magnification views (**B**) from routine screening mammography demonstrate a small, ill-defined mass with minimal spiculation. This was nonpalpable, and biopsy demonstrated infiltrating ductal carcinoma. (*From Specht N: Practical Guide to Diagnostic Imaging, St. Louis, Mosby, 1998.*)

2. Breast Ultrasound

Indications
- Characterization of breast mass/density as cystic or solid (Fig. 1-18)
- Guidance for interventional procedure, cyst aspiration, needle localization, fine-needle aspiration (FNA) or core biopsy, prebiopsy localization
- Evaluation of palpable masses in young patients, those who are pregnant or lactating, or those with a palpable abnormality and negative mammogram
- Confirmation, identification, and characterization of masses/density seen on only one view on mammographic examination
- Evaluation of breast implant integrity

Strengths
- Fast
- Noninvasive
- No ionizing radiation
- Readily available

Weaknesses
- Cannot detect microcalcifications
- Large masses can blend with background pattern, limiting their visibility as discrete entities on ultrasound
- Both benign and malignant solid tumors can have similar appearance

Comments
- Breast ultrasound is not indicated as a screening examination for breast disease or for evaluation of microcalcifications.
- Sensitivity for evaluation of breast implant rupture is 70%, specificity 70%.
- Cost: $

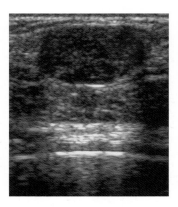

Figure 1-18 High-resolution linear ultrasound image demonstrates an oval, homogeneously hypoechoic mass with characteristics of a probably benign breast mass. *(From Specht N: Practical Guide to Diagnostic Imaging, St. Louis, Mosby, 1998.)*

3. Magnetic Resonance Imaging of the Breast

Indications

- Staging of breast cancer for treatment planning (e.g., detection of chest wall involvement). Preoperative MRI has been shown to detect unsuspected multifocal and multicentric disease in nearly 30% of patients and contralateral disease in up to 5%
- Breast augmentation: evaluation of silicone implant integrity and screening, including patients who have received silicone implants
- Malignant axillary adenopathy with occult primary (Fig. 1-19); useful in patients with positive axillary lymph node for cancer and negative mammogram and ultrasound
- Screening for breast neoplasm in women at high risk (BRCA gene carriers, personal history of breast cancer, strong family history of breast cancer, prior radiation to chest, prior atypical ductal or lobular hyperplasia and lobular carcinoma in situ [LCIS])
- Additional evaluation of contradictory/inconclusive/equivocal mammogram results
- Differentiation between scar tissue and recurrent breast cancer after lumpectomy

Strengths

- More sensitive than mammogram for detecting breast neoplasm; sensitivity 88% to 100%, specificity 30% to 90%
- Sensitivity for breast implant rupture is 94%, specificity 97%

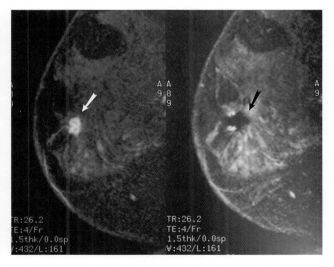

Figure 1-19 MRI-guided wire localization. Images of a patient with malignant axillary adenopathy and unknown primary. Sagittal, fat-suppressed contrast-enhanced three-dimensional FSPGR MRI reveals a peripherally enhancing lesion (arrow in left image) localized by an MRI-compatible needle (arrow in right image). Invasive ductal carcinoma was found at excisional biopsy. *(From Grainger RG, Allison D: Grainger & Allison's Diagnostic Radiology: a Textbook of Medical Imaging, Churchill Livingstone, ed 4, 2001.)*

Weaknesses
- High rate of false positives

Comments
- Breast MRI has emerged as the most sensitive imaging modality for the detection of invasive breast carcinoma; however, it is much more expensive than mammography and is not currently a replacement for screening mammography.
- Scheduling guidelines: When used for additional evaluation of equivocal mammogram, Patients should have recent (within 4 months) mammogram available for correlation.
- Cost: MRI with and without contrast $$$$

C.   Cardiac Imaging

1. Stress Echocardiography

Indications
- Suspected myocardial ischemia based on electrocardiogram (ECG) changes, history
- Post–myocardial infarction (MI), post–coronary artery bypass graft (CABG), post-angioplasty risk stratification
- Evaluation of chest pain in patients with Wolff-Parkinson-White syndrome
- Evaluation of young female with chest pain (high rates of false-positive results with conventional stress test)
- Evaluation of adequacy of therapy while patient is on medication
- Evaluation of patients with significant abnormalities on resting ECG (e.g., left bundle branch block [LBBB] or paced rhythm, left ventricular hypertrophy [LVH] and baseline ST segment or T-wave abnormalities, sloping ST segment secondary to digitalis administration)
- Preoperative risk assessment

Strengths
- Readily available at many institutions (e.g., can be used on weekends or evenings when nuclear testing may be difficult to arrange)
- Useful to detect regional wall abnormalities that occur during myocardial ischemia associated with coronary artery disease
- Significantly higher sensitivity for diagnosing coronary artery disease than conventional treadmill exercise test
- Dobutamine echocardiography is preferable to dipyridamole or adenosine scintigraphy in patients with moderate or severe bronchospastic disease

Weaknesses
- More expensive than conventional treadmill exercise test

Comments
- In stress echocardiography, decrements in contractile function are directly related to decreases in regional subendocardial blood flow.
- Pharmacologic agents (e.g., dobutamine) can be used to induce stress to evaluate cardiac function in selected patients who cannot exercise on a treadmill or bicycle because of orthopedic or other problems.
- When stress echocardiography is used for preoperative assessment, the presence of one or more regional wall motion abnormalities with stress is associated with an increased risk of cardiac complications.
- Contraindications to stress testing are unstable angina with recent rest pain, acute myocarditis or pericarditis, uncompensated congestive heart failure (CHF), uncontrolled hypertension, critical aortic stenosis, untreated life-threatening cardiac arrhythmias, advanced AV block, and severe hypertrophic obstructive cardiomyopathy.
- Cost: $$$

2. Cardiovascular Radionuclide Imaging (Thallium, Sestamibi, Dipyridamole [Persantine] Scan)

Indications
- Suspected myocardial ischemia based on ECG changes, history
- Post-MI, post-CABG, post-angioplasty risk stratification
- Evaluation of chest pain in patients with Wolff-Parkinson-White syndrome
- Evaluation of young female with chest pain (high rates of false-positive results with conventional stress test)
- Evaluation of adequacy of therapy while patient on medication
- Evaluation of patients with significant abnormalities on resting ECG (e.g., LBBB or paced rhythm, LVH and baseline ST segment or T-wave abnormalities, sloping ST segment secondary to digitalis administration)
- Preoperative risk assessment

Strengths
- Useful in patients with underlying bundle branch block or paced rhythm
- Useful in patients with LVH and baseline ST-segment or T-wave abnormalities
- Significantly higher sensitivity for diagnosing coronary artery disease than conventional treadmill exercise test
- Advantages of stress perfusion imaging over stress echocardiography are higher sensitivity, especially for one-vessel coronary artery disease, and better accuracy in evaluating possible ischemia when multiple left ventricular wall motion abnormalities are present

Weaknesses
- Expensive
- Lower sensitivity in women than in men; artifacts due to breast attenuation may affect interpretation of scans in women
- Major disadvantage of ^{99m}-Tc-sestamibi is the need to administer separate stress and rest injections to identify regions of reversible ischemia because of its negligible delayed redistribution over time after single IV injection
- Symmetric three-vessel disease may result in false negative

Comments
- Viable myocardial cells extract the labeled radionuclide from the blood. An absent uptake (cold spot on scan) is an indicator of an absence of blood flow to an area of the myocardium. A fixed defect indicates MI at that site, whereas a defect that reperfuses suggests ischemia.
- Dipyridamole (Persantine) can be used in conjunction with thallium imaging in patients who are unable to exercise adequately on a treadmill or bicycle due to orthopedic or other problems. Dypyridamole injection is followed by thallium injection and subsequent imaging. IV dipyridamole increases coronary flow significantly over the resting level without major change in the heart rate blood pressure product, with less angina, and with less ST depression than with exercise. Dipyridamole may cause bronchospasm and is contraindicated in patients with bronchospastic disease.
- If vasodilating agents are contraindicated, inotropic agents (e.g., dobutamine) can be used instead. They increase myocardial oxygen demand by increasing heart rate, systolic blood pressure, and contractility, and secondarily increase blood flow.
- Newer agents such as sestamibi (Cardiolite, Myoview) are chemically bound to technetium. Advantages are better imaging characteristics, decreased attenuation, and faster imaging (Fig. 1-20). Disadvantages are higher cost and lower sensitivity in detecting viable myocardium compared with thallium.
- Contraindications to stress testing are unstable angina with recent rest pain, acute myocarditis or pericarditis, uncompensated CHF, uncontrolled hypertension,

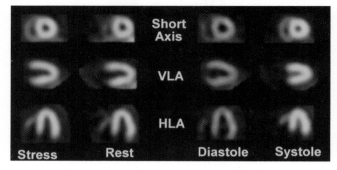

Figure 1-20 Stress and rest SPECT studies (left two columns) in a normal patient, showing representative short-axis, vertical long-axis (VLA), and horizontal long-axis (HLA) images. Note the uniform uptake of ^{99m}Tc-sestamibi on both the stress and the rest tomograms, consistent with homogeneous regional myocardial blood flow. The right two columns show the end-diastolic and end-systolic images acquired during stress and demonstrate uniform systolic thickening in all myocardial segments. The left ventricular cavity size is greater on images acquired during diastole compared with systole, consistent with a normal left ventricular ejection fraction. The "brightness" of the images at end-systole correlates directly with the degree of systolic thickening.   *(From Goldman L, Bennet JC: Cecil Textbook of Medicine, ed 21, Philadelphia, WB Saunders, 2000.)*

critical aortic stenosis, untreated life-threatening cardiac arrhythmias, advanced AV block, and severe hypertrophic obstructive cardiomyopathy.
• Cost: $$$

3. Cardiac MRI (CMR)

Indications
• Evaluation of pericardial effusion
• Constrictive pericarditis (Fig. 1-21)
• Evaluation of distribution of hypertrophy in hypertrophic cardiomyopathy
• Evaluation of right ventricular dysplasia
• Thoracic aorta abnormalities (dissection, coarctation, aneurysm, hematoma)
• Congenital heart disease (intracardiac shunt, anomalous coronary arteries)
• Cardiac neoplasms
• Suspected cardiac involvement from sarcoidosis
• Suspected cardiac hemochromatosis, amyloidosis
• Coronary artery disease (MI, myocardial ischemia)
• Physiologic imaging (bulk flow in large vessels, pressure gradients across stenotic lesions, shunt fraction)
• Quantified cavity volumes, ejection fraction (EF), ventricular mass
• Assessment of bypass grafts (includes magnetic resonance angiography [MRA])

Strengths
• Noninvasive
• No ionizing radiation
• Superior image quality and flexibility in assessment of cardiac anatomy, coronary blood flow, and myocardial perfusion
• Images can be generated in any planar orientation
• Less operator dependent than echocardiogram
• Unlike echocardiography, images are not limited by an acoustic window

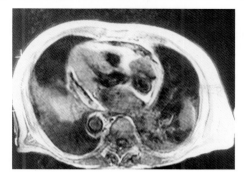

Figure 1-21 MRI of constrictive pericarditis in RA. The dense white infiltrate between the pericardium and gray myocardium is pericardial fluid. *(From Hochberg MC et al, eds: Rheumatology, ed 3, St. Louis, Mosby, 2003.)*

Weaknesses

- Expensive
- Needs cooperative patient
- Time consuming
- Not readily available
- Cannot be performed in patients with non–MR-compatible aneurysm clips, pulmonary artery catheter that includes thermistor wires, pacemaker, cochlear implants, or metallic foreign body in eyes; safe in women with IUDs (including copper ones), and those with surgical clips and staples
- Suboptimal images in patients with irregular rhythm (e.g., atrial fibrillation, frequent ectopy)
- Image distortion in the region immediately surrounding the prosthesis in patients with bioprosthetic and mechanical heart valves
- Image distortion in patients with sternotomy wires and thoracic vascular clips

Comments

- Cardiac magnetic resonance imaging is an excellent imaging technique for evaluation of thoracic aorta and great vessels, cardiac tumors and masses, pericardium and pericardial effusions, and cardiomyopathies and for quantitative assessment of ventricular volumes and mass. Its major limiting factor is its cost disadvantage when compared with ultrasound.
- Myocardial perfusion can be evaluated with MRI by giving an IV contrast agent (e.g., Gd-DPTA), which is taken up by viable myocardial cells concomitantly with dipyridamole or other pharmacologic stress agent.
- Anxious patients (especially those with claustrophobia) should be premedicated with an anxiolytic agent, and their imaging should be done with "open MRI" whenever possible.
- Cost: $$$$

4. Multidetector Computed Tomography

Indications

- This test can be used to identify and measure coronary artery calcifications. Calcification levels can be related to the extent and severity of underlying atherosclerosis and can potentially improve cardiovascular risk prediction. In clinically selected, intermediate-risk patients, it may be reasonable to measure the atherosclerosis burden using multidetector CT to refine clinical risk prediction and to select patients for more aggressive target values for lipid-lowering therapies.

- Coronary calcium measurements are not indicated in patients at low or high risk of cardiovascular disease.
- Multidetector CT is useful in excluding coronary disease in selected patients in whom a false-positive or inconclusive stress test is suspected.
- Coronary calcium assessment may be considered in symptomatic patients to determine the cause of cardiomyopathy.

Strengths
- Speed
- Safety (less invasive than angiography)
- Lower cost than angiography
- High sensitivity and negative predictive value

Weaknesses
- Limited to patients with regular rhythm and slow rates
- Poor images in morbidly obese patients
- Inaccurate visualization of the coronary artery within a stent
- Coronary calcification interferes with images obtained by CT; decreased diagnostic accuracy in older patients due to the prevalence and severity of coronary calcifications with increasing age
- High radiation exposure

Comments
- If calcification is detected in the coronary arteries, a "calcium score" is computed for each of the coronary arteries based upon the size and density of the regions identified to contain calcium. Although the calcium score does not correspond directly to narrowing in the artery due to atherosclerosis, it correlates with the severity of coronary atherosclerosis present. For example, a calcium score of 1 to 10 indicates minimal plaque burden and low likelihood of coronary artery disease, whereas a score of 101 to 400 indicates moderate plaque burden and high likelihood of moderate nonobstructive coronary artery disease. The calcium score can also be used to compare the patient's results with others of the same age and gender to determine a percentile ranking.
- Reasonable test to assess patients who have equivocal treadmill or functional test results, and to assess patients with chest pain who have equivocal or normal echocardiography findings and negative cardiac enzyme results.
- Research data is currently insufficient on the use of serial cardiac CT in assessing subclinical atherosclerosis over time and in detecting noncalcified plaque.
- Cost: $$$$

5. Transesophageal Echocardiogram (TEE)

Indications
- Suspected SBE
- Evaluation of prosthetic valves
- Evaluation of embolic source
- Suspected aortic dissection
- Identification of intracardiac shunts
- Visualization of atrial thrombi
- Diseases of aorta
- Intracardiac mass

Strengths
- Image quality superior to transthoracic echocardiogram (TTE)
- No ionizing radiation

Weaknesses
- Invasive
- Requires patient preparation, monitoring
- Complications rate of 0.2% to 0.5% (e.g., esophageal trauma, aspiration, cardiac dysrhythmias, respiratory depression secondary to sedation)

Comments
- TEE is performed by mounting an ultrasound transducer at the end of a flexible tube to image the heart from the esophagus (Fig. 1-22).
- Useful modality for assessing valvular pathology and diseases of the aorta.
- Cost: $$$

6. Transthoracic Echocardiography

Indications
- Evaluation of heart murmur
- Chest pain

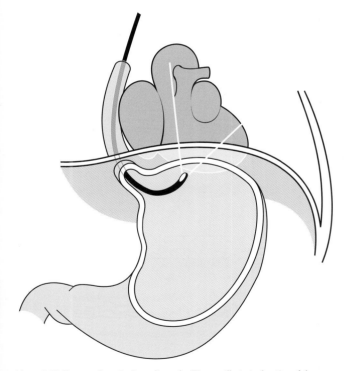

Figure 1-22 Transesophageal echocardiography. Diagram illustrates location of the transesophageal endoscope within the esophagus. *(From Pagana KD, Pagana, TJ: Mosby's Diagnostic and Laboratory Test Reference, ed 8, St. Louis, Mosby, 2007.)*

- Evaluation of ejection fraction
- Systemic embolus
- Syncope of suspected cardiac etiology
- Suspected endocarditis
- Pericardial effusion
- Abnormal heart size on chest film
- Atrial septal defect (ASD)
- Ventricular septal defect (VSD)
- Valvulopathy (Fig. 1-23)
- Cardiomyopathy (Fig. 1-24)
- Guidance of needle placement for pericardiocentesis

Strengths
- Noninvasive
- Fast
- Can be performed at bedside
- No need for patient preparation, premedication, or monitoring
- No ionizing radiation

Weaknesses
- Less sensitive than TEE for SBE, prosthetic valves
- Limited use in obese patients, patients with chronic obstructive pulmonary disease (COPD), those with chest deformities
- Resting echocardiogram not sensitive for detecting coronary artery disease (CAD)

Comments
- TEE is preferred over TTE in evaluation of prosthetic valve, embolic source evaluation, and SBE.

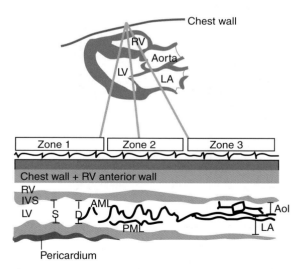

Figure 1-23 Echocardiogram. *(From Weissleder R, Wittenberg J, Harisinghani MG, Chen JW: Primer of Diagnostic Imaging, ed 4, St. Louis, Mosby, 2007.)*

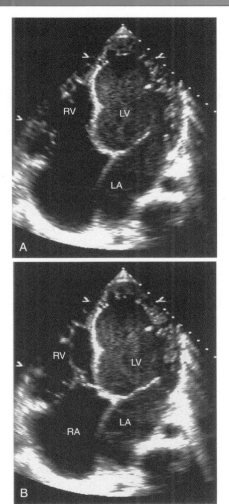

Figure 1-24 Dilated cardiomyopathy. **A**, Diastolic and
B, systolic echocardiographic images demonstrating dilated
cardiomyopathy with severe biventricular systolic dysfunction. Spontaneous contrast is noted in the left ventricle,
consistent with stagnant flow. *LA*, Left atrium; *LV*, left
ventricle; *RA*, right atrium; *RV*, right ventricle. *(From
Crawford, MH, DiMarco JP, Paulus WJ, eds: Cardiology,
ed 2, St. Louis, Mosby, 2004.)*

- Doppler echocardiogram is useful for evaluation of shunts and stenotic or regurgitant valves and for measurement of cardiac output.
- Contrast echocardiography uses commercially produced microbubbles or agitated saline and air to obtain a better definition when evaluating for intracardiac shunts.
- Cost: $$

D.   Chest Imaging

1. Chest Radiograph

Indications
- Dyspnea
- Chest trauma
- Chest pain
- Chronic cough
- Hemoptysis
- Suspected lung neoplasm (primary or metastatic)
- Suspected infectious process (e.g., tuberculosis [TB], pneumonia)
- Inhalation injury
- Pulmonary nodule
- Suspected pleural effusion
- Pneumothorax
- Pulmonary plaques
- Pneumonia follow-up
- Assessment before cardiopulmonary surgery
- Confirmation of feeding tube placement, Swan-Gans catheter, central venous catheter, endotracheal tube, transvenous ventricular pacemaker
- Suspected acute respiratory distress syndrome (ARDS), congestive heart failure (CHF)
- Mesothelioma
- Interstitial lung disease

Strengths
- Low cost
- Readily available
- Low radiation
- Can be performed at bedside

Weaknesses
- Low diagnostic yield
- For portable chest x-radiographs, poor results in obese patients, heart overmagnification due to film taken anteroposteriorly, poor respiratory effort, and poor positioning of patients

Comments
- Proper exposure for evaluating the cardiac structures is present when the spine is just visible behind the heart.
- Radiographs are the most cost-effective method of staging chest pathology.
- Fig. 1-25 describes normal anatomy on chest radiograph.
- Cost: $

2. CT of Chest

Indications
- Nondiagnostic, abnormal plain chest radiograph (e.g., characterization of chest masses, pleural masses, cavitary or cystic changes, or nonspecific infiltrates noted on plain chest films)

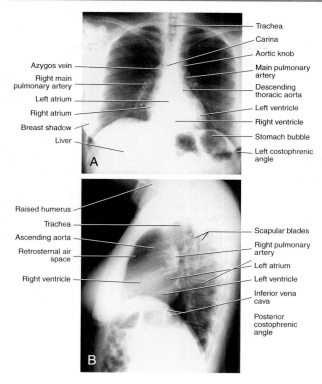

Figure 1-25 Normal anatomy on the female chest radiograph in (**A**) the upright posteroanterior projection and (**B**) the lateral projection. *(From Mettler FA: Primary Care Radiology, Philadelphia, WB Saunders, 2000.)*

- Follow-up of pulmonary nodule
- Staging of lung carcinoma
- Mediastinal widening
- Evaluation of bronchiectasis and interstitial lung disease
- Chest trauma
- Characterization of suspected thoracic aortic pathology
- Abnormal hilum
- Differentiation of pleural from parenchymal abnormalities
- Evaluation of thymus in patients with myasthenia gravis
- Suspicion of aortic dissection (Fig. 1-26)

Strengths
- Fast
- Preferred method for examining the hila and the mediastinum
- Excellent method for evaluation of pleura and chest wall

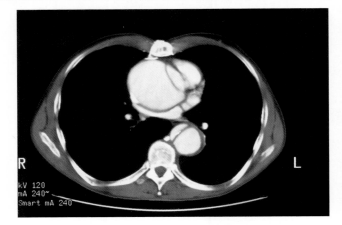

Figure 1-26 Spiral CT in acute type A dissection extending into the descending aorta. The ascending aorta is dilated. The intimal flap is clearly seen in both the ascending and descending aorta. Courtesy of Dr. Loren Ketai, University of New Mexico, USA. *(From Crawford, MH, DiMarco JP, Paulus WJ, eds: Cardiology, ed 2, St. Louis, Mosby, 2004.)*

Weaknesses
- Potential for significant contrast reaction
- Expensive
- Radiation exposure

Comments
- Contrast enhancement may be necessary for the evaluation of known or suspected vascular abnormalities (e.g., aortic aneurysm or dissection), abnormal hilum, and certain abnormalities of the pleura.
- High-resolution chest CT uses a specific algorithm of very thin slices to evaluate for interstitial lung diseases, bronchiectasis, or lymphangitic spread of carcinoma.
- Cost: $ CT of chest without contrast $$$; CT of chest with and without contrast $$$$

3. Helical (Spiral) CT of Chest

Indications
- Evaluation of solitary pulmonary nodule for densitometry
- Detection of metastatic disease
- Detection of pulmonary embolism (PE)
- Evaluation of peridiaphragmatic lesions
- Evaluation of airways and vascular lesions

Strengths
- Permits imaging of chest structures without misregistration due to respiratory motion
- Fast
- Can differentiate acute from chronic pulmonary embolism (PE)
- When used to diagnose PE, can lead to or support alternate diagnosis to explain patient's symptoms
- Good interobserver agreement
- Optimal initial test for PE in patient with abnormal baseline chest radiograph

Weaknesses

- Potential for significant contrast reaction
- Requires patient cooperation (breath-holding for 10-30 seconds)
- When used to diagnose PE, results can be affected by vena cava obstruction (improper scan delay), shunts (e.g., patent foramen ovale, left-to-right cardiac shunts)
- Can miss subsegmental PE
- Hilar lymphadenopathy or other mediastinal soft tissue masses can mimic PE
- Radiation exposure

Comments

- Helical CT acquires data continuously as the patient is transported through the scanner during a single breathhold.
- Contrast media may be used for the detection of pulmonary thromboembolism.
- Normal spiral CT scan does not rule out PE; sensitivity range is 53% to 100%, specificity 78% to 100%.
- Cost: CT without contrast $$; CT with contrast $$$; CT with and without contrast $$$$

4. MRI of Chest

Indications

- Evaluation of chest wall disease when CT is inconclusive
- Assessment for aortic dissection (Fig. 1-27)
- Assessment of hilar and mediastinal pathology when CT is inconclusive
- Superior sulcus carcinoma
- Posterior mediastinal masses
- Follow-up lymphoma
- Brachial plexus lesions
- Contraindications to contrast medium in patients with mediastinal or vascular abnormality

Strengths

- Noninvasive
- Safe contrast agent
- No ionizing radiation
- Soft tissue resolution
- Multiplanar
- Excellent imaging of mediastinum and chest wall

Weaknesses

- Expensive
- Needs cooperative patient
- Time consuming
- Motion artifacts secondary to cardiac and respiratory movements
- Inadequate imaging of lung (normal lung does not produce an MR signal because of magnetic susceptibility effects)
- Cannot be performed in patients with non–MR-compatible aneurysm clips, pacemaker, cochlear implants, or metallic foreign body in eyes; however, safe in women with IUDs (including copper ones) and those with surgical clips and staples

Comments

- Used predominantly as a problem-solving tool if CT is inconclusive.
- Anxious patients (especially those with claustrophobia) should be premedicated with an anxiolytic agent, and their imaging should be done with "open MRI" whenever possible.
- Cost: MRI with contrast $$$$; MRI without contrast $$$; MRI with and without contrast $$$$$

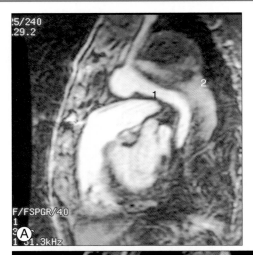

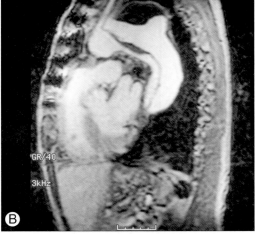

Figure 1-27 Longitudinal MRI in a chronic type B dissection extending into the arch. **A,** Early phase showing (1) the entry point and (2) a faint visualization of the outline of the aneurysm. **B,** Late phase demonstrating partial opacification of the aneurysm and the extension of the dissection along the subclavian artery. *Courtesy of Dr. Loren Ketai, University of New Mexico. (From Crawford, MH, DiMarco JP, Paulus WJ, eds: Cardiology, ed 2, St. Louis, Mosby, 2004.)*

1. Adrenal Medullary Scintigraphy (Metaiodobenzylguanidine [MIBG] Scan)

Indications
- Evaluation of suspected intra-adrenal paraganglioma or pheochromocytoma (Fig. 1-28)
- Survey of the entire body for the presence of extra-adrenal and metastatic lesions from paragangliomas or pheochromocytomas

Strengths
- Sensitivity for detection of pheochromocytoma is greater than 90%, specificity greater than 95%

Weaknesses
- Interference from several drugs (e.g., tricyclic antidepressants, labetolol, cocaine, reserpine) and barium

Comments
- Adrenal medullary scintigraphy uses the tracer metaiodobenzylguanidine (MIBG), an analogue of guanethidine. Uptake occurs in the adrenal medulla, neuroblastic tumor tissues, and other organs with rich adrenergic innervation (e.g., heart, spleen). Commonly used radiolabels are I-131 and I-123. When using I-131 MIGB, initial images are usually obtained at 24 hours and delayed images at 48 and 72 hours after injection. When using I-123 MIGB, initial images are obtained at 2 to 3 hours, delayed ones at 24 and 48 hours.
- Paragangliomas or pheochromocytoma demonstrate unilateral focal uptake.
- Scintigraphy with MIBG should not be used as a screening procedure for pheochromocytoma. MIGB Scintigraphy is indicated only after biochemical tests suggest the diagnosis.
- Additional imaging modalities for pheochromocytoma of adrenal glands are CT and MRI. Both modalities can detect up to 90% of functional tumors.
- Cost: $$

2. Parathyroid Scan

Indications
- Hypercalcemia with elevated parathyroid (PTH) level
- Presurgical localization of source of PTH production

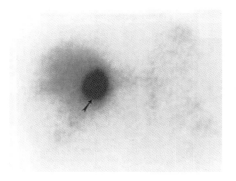

Figure 1-28 Anterior abdominal view on ^{123}I-MIBG scan (72 hours postinjection) of a right adrenal pheochromocytoma *(arrow)*. *(From Besser CM, Thorner MO: Comprehensive Clinical Endocrinology, ed 3, Mosby, 2002.)*

Strengths
- Noninvasive
- Best test to rule out parathyroid adenoma (Fig. 1-29)

Weaknesses
- Parathyroid hyperplasia may result in nondiagnostic scan.
- Recent ingestion of iodine (food, meds) or recent tests with iodine content may interfere with interpretation of results.
- Pregnancy is a relative contraindication.

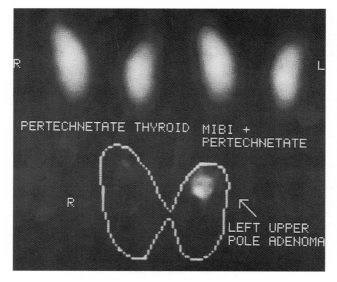

Figure 1-29 Imaging of a parathyroid adenoma. **A,** Pertechnetate thyroid scan obtained conventionally 10 to 20 minutes after the intravenous injection of ^{99m}Tc pertechnetate through an indwelling needle. **B,** Without the patient moving, ^{99m}Tc methoxyisobutylisonitrile (MIBI) is injected and a further series of images is taken. ^{99m}Tc MIBI is taken up both by the parathyroid adenoma and by normal thyroid so that a combined composite image is seen. Using a change detection algorithm, the change between the two images is determined and the statistical degree of that difference is plotted as a probability. **C,** The higher intensity in the upper pole of the left lobe of the thyroid indicated a change between the two images with a significance of over 1 in 1000. This is the site of the upper-pole parathyroid adenoma. The outline of the thyroid is also shown. A small area of increased probability of change is also seen in the upper-pole thyroid adenoma was removed, and a right upper-pole hyperplastic gland (100 mg) was also removed. Before imaging, it is important biochemically to confirm that hypercalcemia is due to hyperparathyroidism. Imaging of the parathyroid is intended to localize the site of adenomas or hyperplastic glands. Visualization of a gland depends upon its size. A normal parathyroid gland of less than 20 mg will not be visualized by this technique. Earlier attempts to image parathyroid glands using thallium in a similar way have proved less successful than the use of MIBI. *(From Besser CM, Thorner MO: Comprehensive Clinical Endocrinology, ed 3, Mosby, 2002.)*

Comments
- It is necessary to look for an ectopic location in the chest or other location in the neck when evaluating a parathyroid scan.
- Cost: $$

3. Thyroid Scan (Radioiodine Uptake Study)

Indications
- Thyroiditis
- Hyperthyroidism
- Thyroid nodule (Fig. 1-30)
- Detection of lingual thyroid
- Thyroglossal cyst

Strengths
- Noninvasive

Weaknesses
- Contraindicated in pregnancy because radioiodine crosses the placenta; significant exposure of the fetal thyroid can occur and may result in cretinism.
- Radioiodine is excreted in human breast milk. Nursing should be stopped following diagnostic studies with radioiodine
- Significant interference from iodine contained in foods and medications can interfere with imaging.

Comments
- In the normal euthyroid subject, distribution of radiotracer is homogeneous and uniform throughout the gland.
- In Graves' disease, concentration of activity is uniformly increased.
- In Hashimoto's disease, radioiodine uptake values are variable depending on the stage of disease.

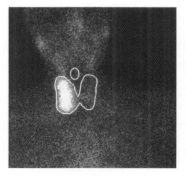

Figure 1-30 A 131I scan demonstrates an area of increased uptake in the right lobe of a 32-year-old woman with increased thyroid function tests and a palpable nodule. This scan is consistent with a toxic or hyperfunctioning nodule. *(From Townsend CM, Beauchamp RD, Evers BM, Mattox KL, eds: Sabiston Textbook of Surgery, ed 17, Philadelphia, Saunders, 2004.)*

- In nontoxic nodular goiter, several areas experience relatively increased activity and in other areas activity is decreased.
- In toxic hot nodule, a rounded area of markedly increased concentration of activity is seen.
- Cost: $$

4. Thyroid Ultrasound

Indications
- Thyroid nodule(s) (Fig. 1-31)
- Thyromegaly
- Multinodular goiter
- Parathyroid abnormalities
- To direct image-guided biopsy

Strengths
- Noninvasive
- Fast
- No ionizing radiation

Weaknesses
- Fine-needle aspiration biopsy necessary for definitive diagnosis
- May miss nodules less than 1 cm in diameter
- Interpretation of large cysts (>4 cm) often difficult due to presence of areas of cystic or hemorrhagic degeneration

Comments
- Ultrasound is an excellent modality to demonstrate thyroid gland anatomy and to guide biopsy or cyst aspiration.
- Thyroid ultrasound is also useful to detect parathyroid abnormalities.
- Approximately 70% of parathyroid lesions are evident on ultrasound.
- Cost: $

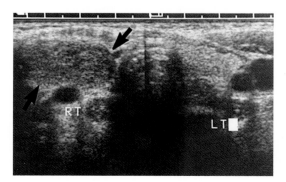

Figure 1-31 Preoperative ultrasound of a patient with a 4- × -2-cm homogeneous right thyroid *(RT)* mass *(arrows)*. Resection demonstrated a follicular adenoma. *LT,* left thyroid. *(From Townsend CM, Beauchamp RD, Evers BM, Mattox KL, eds: Sabiston Textbook of Surgery, ed 17, Philadelphia, Saunders, 2004.)*

1. Obstetric Ultrasound

Indications
- Determination of gestational age (size/date discrepancy ≥2 weeks, before elective pregnancy termination)
- Multiple gestation (determination of fetal number)
- Suspected fetal demise
- Suspected abortion
- Incomplete abortion
- Spontaneous abortion
- Determination of fetal presentation
- Fetal anatomy survey
- Placental evaluation
- Diagnosis of fetal abnormalities
- Umbilical cord evaluation
- Vaginal bleeding
- Suspected congenital abnormality
- Assistance in obtaining amniotic fluid
- Maternal disease (e.g., hypertension, diabetes mellitus, rubella, cytomegalovirus [CMV], human immunodeficiency virus [HIV])
- Preterm labor or rupture of membranes before 36 weeks
- Suspected placental abruption
- First-degree relative with congenital anomaly
- Evaluate for fetal growth and for intrauterine growth retardation (IUGR)

Strengths
- Fast
- Noninvasive
- Readily available
- No ionizing radiation
- Can be repeated serially

Weaknesses
- 20% false negative rate in ectopic pregnancy
- May miss placental abruption if there is no retroplacental hemorrhage at time of scan or inadequate visualization of hemorrhage; blood may be isoechoic to placenta and difficult to evaluate

Comments
- Cost: $$

2. Pelvic Ultrasound

Indications
- Pelvic mass
- Pelvic pain
- Infertility
- Uterine/ovarian mass
- Uterine (Müllerian) anomalies
- Pregnancy, including ectopic
- Abnormal vaginal bleeding

Strengths
- Fast
- Can be performed at bedside
- Low cost
- Noninvasive
- No radiation

- No need for contrast agent
- Examination not affected by renal function
- Readily available

Weaknesses
- Shadowing by gas, bone, or calculi often obscures views behind acoustic shadowing
- Ultrasonographic studies are operator dependent
- Affected by body habitus
- Requires patient cooperation and full bladder

Comments
- Typically consists of transabdominal and transvaginal scanning
- Cost: $$

3. Prostate Ultrasound

Indications
- Guidance for biopsy (Fig. 1-32)
- Abnormal digital rectal examination
- Voiding difficulty
- Elevated prostate-specific antigen (PSA)
- Infertility workup

Strengths
- No ionizing radiation
- Imaging modality of choice as a guide to needle biopsy in suspected prostate carcinoma
- Useful to assess bladder volume and estimate size of prostate

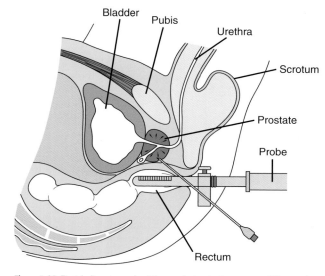

Figure 1-32 Rectal ultrasonography. Diagram demonstrating transrectal biopsy of the prostate. *(From Pagana KD, Pagana, TJ: Mosby's Diagnostic and Laboratory Test Reference, ed 8, St. Louis, Mosby, 2007.)*

Weaknesses
- Invasive and uncomfortable for patients
- Fecal material in rectum will interfere with sonogram results

Comments
- Cost: $$

4. Renal Ultrasound

Indications
- Renal insufficiency
- Nephrolithiasis
- Renal mass
- Polycystic kidney disease
- Acquired cystic renal disease
- Hydronephrosis
- Pyelonephritis
- Renal infarction
- Acute/chronic renal failure

Strengths
- Noninvasive
- Can be performed at bedside
- Fast
- No ionizing radiation
- Readily available

Weaknesses
- Affected by body habitus
- Retained barium from radiographs may interfere with results

Comments
- Cost: $$

5. Scrotal Ultrasound

Indications
- Testicular pain or swelling
- Testicular trauma
- Testicular or other scrotal masses
- Search for undescended testicle
- Infertility evaluation
- Testicular torsion
- Infection

Strengths
- Noninvasive
- Fast
- Requires no patient preparation
- No ionizing radiation

Weaknesses
- Not useful for staging of testicular neoplasm (MRI is preferred)

Comments
- Color Doppler ultrasound is the imaging modality of choice when suspecting testicular torsion; however, nuclear medicine flow study can also be used for diagnosis.
- Cost: $

6. Tranvaginal (Endovaginal) Ultrasound

Indications
- Evaluation of adenexa/ovaries
- Evaluation of pregnancy
- Infertility workup
- Suspected ectopic pregnancy
- Suspected endometrial abnormalities (Fig. 1-33)
- Guidance for aspiration/biopsy of pelvic fluid collection/mass
- Lost IUD

Strengths
- Useful for evaluation of obese or gaseous patients
- Very good resolution images of pelvis
- No ionizing radiation
- Full bladder not required
- Earlier detection of pregnancy when compared with transabdominal ultrasound

Weaknesses
- Unable to evaluate false pelvis
- Limited field of view secondary to high-frequency transducer
- Will miss any structures/abnormalities more than 10 cm away from transducer

Comments
- Contraindications include imperforate hymen, patient refusal, premature membrane rupture (increased risk of infection)
- Cost: $$

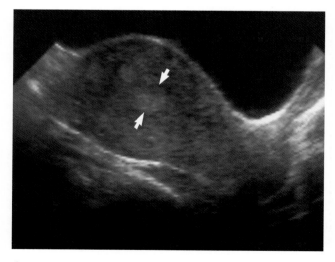

Figure 1-33 Transvaginal ultrasound. The endometrium appears thickened and irregular *(arrows)* in this patient with endometrial cancer. *(From Grainger RG, Allison D: Grainger & Allison's Diagnostic Radiology: A Textbook of Medical Imaging, Churchill Livingstone, ed 4, 2001.)*

7. Urinary Bladder Ultrasound

Indications
- Hematuria
- Recurrent cystitis
- Bladder neoplasm (primary or metastatic)
- Urinary incontinence
- Bladder diverticuli
- Bladder calculi
- Evaluation of masses posterior to the bladder

Strengths
- Noninvasive
- Fast
- No ionizing radiation
- Can be performed at bedside

Weaknesses
- Affected by overlying bowel gas and body habitus (e.g., in morbidly obese patient, fat overlying bladder impedes visualization)
- Operator dependent; results may be affected by skill of technician
- Requires cooperative patient and full bladder distention

Comments
- Cost: $$

8. Hysterosalpingography (HSG)

Indications
- Primary and secondary infertility
- Diagnosis of tubal anomalies (including diverticula and accessory ostia) (Fig. 1-34)
- Evaluate tube patency after tubal ligation

Strengths
- Less expensive than laparoscopy
- Rapid (takes 10 minutes to perform) and relatively safe (complications occur in less than 3% of patients)

Weaknesses
- Limited diagnostic use (discovers only 50% of peritubal disease diagnosed by direct visualization via laparoscope)
- Can result in pain, infection, and contrast allergy

Comments
- HSG is an imaging modality in which the uterine cavity and the lumina of the fallopian tubes are visualized by injecting contrast material through the cervical canal.
- Contraindications to HSG are acute pelvic infection, pregnancy, active uterine bleeding, recent uterine surgery, and allergy to iodine.
- HSG should be performed only on days 6 to 12 after last menstrual period (LMP).
- Cost: $$

9. Intravenous Pyelography (IVP) and Retrograde Pyelography

Indications
- Hematuria
- Suspected urolithiasis
- Renal cell carcinoma
- Renal and ureteral anomalies, strictures
- Bladder tumors, diverticuli, cystocele, calculi

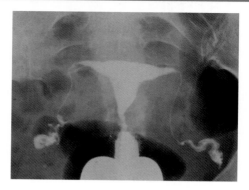

Figure 1-34 A normal hysterosalpingogram. The triangular outline of the uterine cavity is seen, with passage of dye along the fallopian tubes and spill into the peritoneal cavity. *(From Greer IA, Cameron IT, Kitchener HC, Prentice A: Mosby's Color Atlas and Text of Obstetrics and Gynecology, London, Harcourt, 2001.)*

- Enterovesical fistulas (e.g., Crohn's disease, diverticulitis, trauma, surgery)
- Retrograde urethrogram mainly used for evaluation of strictures or anterior urethral disease in males and to confirm equivocal findings on IVP

Strengths
- Inexpensive
- Provides both functional and anatomic information (may identify anatomic abnormalities that predispose to stone formation)
- Able to image entire urinary tract
- Shows precise site of obstruction in urolithiasis

Weaknesses
- Potential for significant IV contrast reaction
- Gas in the rectum can mimic filling defect in bladder
- Requires patient preparation to minimize intestinal gas and feces, which may mask abnormal findings
- Contraindicated in pregnancy
- Examination affected by renal function
- Compression of proximal bulbar urethra by prominent bulbocavernous muscles may be mistaken for urethral stricture
- Retained barium from previous barium examination can interfere with interpretation
- Radiation exposure

Comments
- Ultrasonography and CT have largely replaced IVP as the initial studies in urologic imaging during the last two decades.
- Risk of contrast-induced nephrotoxicity is 3% to 7%. Increased risk in patients with dehydration, diabetes mellitus (DM), and creatinine 1.4 mg/dl or higher.
- Increased risk of contrast reaction in patients with prior reaction, history of asthma, or severe allergies. Risk of IV contrast reaction is much lower when using nonionic contrast; however, nonionic contrast is much more expensive.
- Cost: $$

1. Plain X-Ray Films of Skeletal System

Indications
• Trauma
• Infections (osteomyelitis, TB)
• Scoliosis and other developmental abnormalities
• Rheumatoid arthritis (RA) (Fig. 1-35), psoriatic arthritis, ankylosing spondylitis, Reiter's syndrome
• Paget's disease of bone
• Compression fractures
• Osteoarthritis
• Tumor-like processes (fibrous dysplasia, bony cysts)
• Bone neoplasms (primary or metastatic)
• Bone pain
• Multiple myeloma
• Legg-Calvé-Perthes syndrome
• Osgood-Schlatter's disease
• Gout
• Hyperthyroidism
• Hemochromatosis

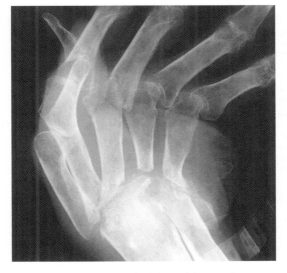

Figure 1-35 Metacarpophalangeal (MCP) joint deformities. Severe ulnar deviation at the MCP joints is associated with osseous erosions of the metacarpal heads. Observe complete destruction of the wrist, with resorption of the carpal bones and bases of the metacarpal bones. Osseous defects are observed at the distal radius and ulna. Radial deviation of the wrist associated with ulnar deviation of the MCP joints has produced a "zigzag" deformity. *(From Hochberg MC et al, eds: Rheumatology, ed 3, St. Louis, Mosby, 2003.)*

- Evaluation of bone alignment
- Evaluate prosthesis

Strengths
- Inexpensive
- Readily available

Weaknesses
- May miss stress fractures
- May miss aseptic vascular necrosis
- May miss early osteomyelitis, septic arthritis

Comments
- Cost: $

2. Bone Densitometry (Dual-Energy X-Ray Absorptiometry [DEXA] Scan)

Indications
- Postmenopausal women 65 years or older, regardless of additional risk factors
- Postmenopausal women younger than 65 years and with additional risk factors for osteoporotic fractures (parental history of hip fracture, current cigarette smoking, a body weight less than 58 kg, use [or plans to use] corticosteroids longer than 3 months, or serious long-term conditions thought to increase fracture risk, such as hyperthyroidism or malabsorption)
- Follow-up hormone therapy

Strengths
- Readily available
- Noninvasive
- Faster and less radiation than quantitative computed tomography (QCT)
- Can be performed serially to assess disease progression

Weaknesses
- Less sensitive than QCT for detecting early trabecular bone loss

Comments
- The decision to test for bone mineral density (BMD) should be based on an individual's risk profile, and testing is never indicated unless the results are likely to influence a treatment decision.
- Bone density measurement at a specific skeletal site predicts fractures at that site better than bone density measurements made at a different skeletal site.
- Cost: $$

3. MRI of Spine

Indications
- Suspected neoplasm (primary or metastatic)
- Radiculopathy
- Acute myelopathy
- New or progressive neurologic deficit
- High-impact trauma
- Suspected spinal infection
- Neurogenic claudication (onset with prolonged standing, relief with back flexion)
- Spinal hematoma
- Syringohydromyelia
- Failure of conservative therapy for back pain
- Spinal stenosis
- Back pain in patient with cancer

Strengths
- Noninvasive
- Safe contrast agent (MRI uses gadolinium, an IV agent that is not nephrotoxic)
- No ionizing radiation
- Soft tissue resolution
- Multiplanar
- Best for identifying disk changes and evaluating extent of injury
- Excellent modality for evaluation of intradural metastases and intramedullary tumors

Weaknesses
- Expensive
- Needs cooperative patient
- Time consuming
- Cannot be performed in patients with non–MR-compatible aneurysm clips, pacemaker, cochlear implants, or metallic foreign body in eyes; safe in women with IUDs (including copper ones), and those with surgical clips and staples

Comments
- Imaging for back pain should generally only be considered after conservative management fails. Exceptions are back pain with neurologic symptoms (e.g., sphincter disturbances, reflex changes), HIV infection, IV drug use, and history of cancer.
- The sensitivity and specificity of MRI for disk herniations is similar to that of myelography; however, MRI is the best imaging test for suspected lateral disk herniation because of its multiplanar capabilities
- For evaluation of intra-axial and extra-axial spinal lesions, MR is the procedure of choice due to its high soft-tissue resolution and multilinear capabilities.
- MRI is the procedure of choice in patients with suspected spinal stenosis.
- Enhanced images are indicated when infection, inflammation, neoplasia, intrinsic spinal cord lesions, or extradural spinal cord lesions from primary neoplastic or metastatic lesions are suspected or after spinal surgery to separate scar from recurrent disk.
- Unenhanced images are indicated in suspected degenerative disease of spine and spinal cord trauma.
- May be of limited use after back surgery because of metallic artifact from hardware.
- Anxious patients (especially those with claustrophobia) should be premedicated with an anxiolytic agent, and their imaging should be done with "open MRI" whenever possible.
- Cost: MRI without contrast $$$$; MRI with and without contrast $$$$$

4. MRI of Shoulder

Indications
- Rotator cuff tear (Fig. 1-36)
- Glenohumeral dislocation
- Glenoid labral tear
- Persistent shoulder pain despite conservative treatment when shoulder surgery is contemplated

Strengths
- Sensitivity and specificity for suspected rotator cuff tears is 85% for partial tears; 95% for full tear
- Sensitivity for suspected glenoid labral tear is greater than 90% (same as arthrography)

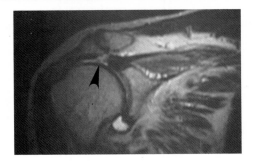

Figure 1-36 MRI of complete rotator-cuff tear. T2-weighted MR image of the shoulder shows discontinuity of the supraspinatus tendon indicative of complete tear *(arrow)*. The proximal tendon margin is frayed and retracted 1.5 cm. Focal swelling and increased signal in opposing articular cartilages of the glenohumeral joint are evidence of early degenerative disease. *(From Hochberg MC et al, eds: Rheumatology, ed 3, St. Louis, Mosby, 2003.)*

Weaknesses
- Expensive
- Needs cooperative patient
- Time consuming
- Cannot be performed in patients with non–MR-compatible aneurysm clips, pacemaker, cochlear implants, or metallic foreign body in eyes; safe in women with IUDs (including copper ones), and those with surgical clips and staples

Comments
- Excellent imaging modality for evaluation of cartilage, tendons, ligaments, and soft tissue abnormalities.
- Anxious patients (especially those with claustrophobia) should be premedicated with an anxiolytic agent, and their imaging should be done with "open MRI" whenever possible.
- Cost: MRI without contrast $$$$

5. MRI of Hip

Indications
- Aseptic necrosis of hip
- Nondisplaced hip fracture
- Legg-Calvé-Perthes disease
- Hip pain with negative plain films
- Transient osteoporosis of the hip
- Suspected neoplasm
- Suspected osteomyelitis

Strengths
- Most sensitive imaging modality for early aseptic necrosis

Weaknesses
- Expensive
- Needs cooperative patient
- Time consuming

- Cannot be performed in patients with non–MR-compatible aneurysm clips, pacemaker, cochlear implants, or metallic foreign body in eyes; safe in women with IUDs (including copper ones), and those with surgical clips and staples

Comments
- Excellent imaging modality for evaluation of cartilage, tendons, ligaments, and soft tissue abnormalities.
- Anxious patients (especially those with claustrophobia) should be premedicated with an anxiolitic agent, and their imaging should be done with "open MRI" whenever possible.
- Cost: $$$$

6. MRI of Pelvis

Indications
- Leiomyoma location
- Endometriosis
- Adenomyosis
- Congenital abnormalities
- Presurgical planning
- Suspected neoplasm
- Suspected osteomyelitis

Strengths
- Noninvasive
- Safe contrast agent (MRI uses gadolinium, an IV agent that is less nephrotoxic)
- No ionizing radiation

Weaknesses
- Expensive
- Needs cooperative patient
- Time consuming
- Cannot be performed in patients with non–MR-compatible aneurysm clips, pacemaker, cochlear implants, or metallic foreign body in eyes; safe in women with IUDs (including copper ones), and those with surgical clips and staples

Comments
- Anxious patients (especially those with claustrophobia) should be premedicated with an anxiolitic agent, and their imaging should be done with "open MRI" whenever possible.
- Cost: $$$$

7. MRI of Knee

Indications
- Cruciate ligament tear
- Medial collateral ligament tear
- Meniscal tear
- Patellar dislocation/fracture
- Loose body
- Occult knee fracture
- Septic arthritis (Fig. 1-37)

Strengths
- Excellent imaging modality for evaluation of cartilage, tendons, ligaments, and soft tissue abnormalities

Weaknesses
- Expensive
- Needs cooperative patient

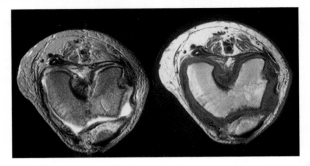

Figure 1-37 MRI scan of right knee of a patient who has *Staphylococcus aureus* septic arthritis. Note the soft tissue inflammation and a joint effusion. *(From Cohen J, Powderly WG: Infectious Diseases, ed 2, St. Louis, Mosby, 2004.)*

- Time consuming
- Cannot be performed in patients with non–MR-compatible aneurysm clips, pacemaker, cochlear implants, or metallic foreign body in eyes; safe in women with IUDs (including copper ones), and those with surgical clips and staples

Comments
- MRI is not indicated when physical examination is unequivocal. It should be performed only when physical examination is inconclusive or equivocal and the physician strongly suspects a tear or other significant abnormalities.
- Anxious patients (especially those with claustrophobia) should be premedicated with an anxiolitic agent, and their imaging should be done with "open MRI" whenever possible.
- Cost: MRI without contrast $$$

8. CT of Spinal Cord

Indications
- Radiculopathy
- Intervertebral disk disease
- Spondylolisthesis
- Primary or metastatic spinal cord neoplasms
- Spinal nerve tumors
- Syringohydromyelia
- High-impact trauma
- Infection

Strengths
- Fast
- Easy to monitor patients
- Useful to identify difficult anatomic regions not well visualized by plain films (e.g., C1-C2, C7-T1)

Weaknesses
- Potential for significant contrast reaction
- Less sensitive than MRI in identifying intrinsic damage to the spinal cord, extrinsic compression, and ligamentous injury

Comments
- Imaging for back pain should generally only be considered after conservative management fails. Exceptions are back pain with neurologic symptoms (e.g., sphincter disturbances, reflex changes), HIV infection, IV drug use, and history of cancer.
- Enhanced images are indicated when infection, inflammation, neoplasia, intrinsic spinal cord lesions, or extradural spinal cord lesions from primary neoplastic or metastatic lesions are suspected and after spinal surgery to separate scar from recurrent disk.
- Unenhanced images are indicated in suspected degenerative disease of spine and spinal cord trauma
- Cost: $$$

9. Arthrography

Indications
- Cartilage injury
- Implant loosening
- Ligament and tendon tears
- Suspected intra-articular loose body

Strengths
- Excellent visualization of ligament, tendon, cartilage injury in shoulder, knee, elbow, wrist, hip, and ankle

Weaknesses
- Invasive
- Potential reaction to contrast media
- Expensive

Comments
- Arthrography is contraindicated in patients with a history of reaction to contrast media or skin infection at the site of injection.
- Cost: CT arthrogram $$$, MRI arthrogram $$$$

10. CT Myelography

Indications
- Evaluation of spinal vascular malformations
- Evaluation of suspected spine lesions (e.g., small osteophytes impinging upon nerve roots)

Strengths
- Excellent for evaluation of small osteophytic lesions and nerve roots
- Can visualize bony stenosis

Weaknesses
- Invasive
- Poor visualization of intramedullary lesions
- Poor soft tissue resolution
- Side effects (e.g., hypersensitivity reactions, headaches, seizures, aseptic meningitis, nausea; headaches in approximately 10% to 25% of patients)

Comments
- This imaging modality is now less commonly used with general availability of MRI. If the patient cannot have an MRI or the MRI is limited (e.g., after spinal fusion), myelogram is the next study of choice.

- Imaging for back pain should generally only be considered after conservative management fails. Exceptions are back pain with neurologic symptoms (e.g., sphincter disturbances, reflex changes), HIV infection, IV drug use, and history of cancer.
- CT myelography is the radiographic examination of the spinal canal and spinal cord with nonionic contrast injected in the subarachnoid space via lumbar puncture or occasionally lateral cervical puncture at C1-C2 level.
- Cost: $$$$

11. Nuclear Imaging (Bone Scan, Gallium Scan, White Blood Cell [WBC] Scan)

Indications
- Infection
- Metastatic disease
- Unexplained bone pain
- Avascular necrosis
- Evaluation of bone lesions seen on other imaging studies
- Seronegative spondyloarthropathies
- Paget's disease of bone
- Metabolic bone diseases (e.g., osteomalacia, hypervitaminosis A or D)
- Assessment of bone graft viability
- Stress fractures/shin splints
- Temporomandibular joint (TMJ) derangement
- Prosthetic loosening
- Reflex sympathetic dystrophy

Strengths
- Highly sensitive for bone lesions
- Three-phase bone imaging is very useful in suspected infection, osteonecrosis, and stress fractures. Gallium and WBC scans can also be performed to look for infection (Figs. 1-38, 1-39).

Weaknesses
- Nonspecific
- Requires availability of current plain bone radiographs for side-by-side comparison
- "Flare phenomenon"—apparent worsening of serial bone scans yet clinical improvement after chemotherapy often seen with metastatic breast and prostate carcinoma due to chemotherapy-related tumor suppression
- Expensive
- Less specific than MRI for osteomyelitis
- False negative scans in multiple myeloma (better detectability with plain radiograph than with radionuclide scan)

Comments
- In bone scanning, a diphosphonate compound (methyldiphosphonate [MDP]) is labeled (e.g., with Tc-99m), becomes incorporated into the mineral phase of bone, and is used to demonstrate bone pathology. The major factors affecting the uptake of the tracer are osteoblastic activity and blood flow.
- *Total body bone imaging* should be performed when suspected disease may involve more than one site.
- *Three-phase bone imaging* is recommended for evaluation of localized area when detection of regional hyperemia is crucial to diagnosis. Common indications are infection, assessment of bone graft viability, and reflex sympathetic dystrophy.

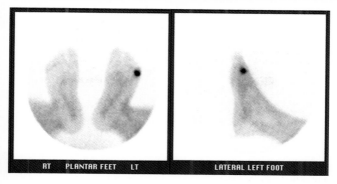

Figure 1-38 Osteomyelitis. Intense accumulation of Tc-99m WBC in the proximal phalanx of the fifth digit of the left foot at 4 hours postinjection. *(From Specht N: Practical Guide to Diagnostic Imaging, St. Louis, Mosby, 1998.)*

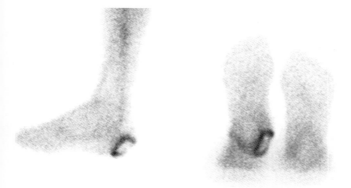

Figure 1-39 Cellulitis. Intense accumulation of Tc-99m WBC outlining margin of heel ulcer but not in bone. *(From Specht N: Practical Guide to Diagnostic Imaging, St. Louis, Mosby, 1998.)*

- *Single-photon emission computed tomography (SPECT) bone imaging* should be requested when a lesion in lumbar spine, knees, skull, or facial bones is suspected. It can also be performed on children to evaluate for spondylolysis.
- Bone scintigraphy should precede CT with contrast when both studies are requested because contrast for CT can affect bone images.
- Cost: limited to one area $$; whole body bone scan $$$

1. CT of Brain

Indications

- Head trauma
- Suspected subarachnoid hemorrhage
- Central nervous system (CNS) neoplasm
- Cerebral hemorrhage
- Cerebral infarct
- Suspected subdural or epidural hematoma
- Hypoxic encephalopathy
- Cranial nerve tumors
- Cerebral imaging in patients with contraindications to MRI (e.g., pacemaker, metallic foreign body)

Strengths

- Fast
- Can easily detect acute parenchymal/subarachnoid hemorrhage and calcifications
- Easy to monitor patients
- Noncontrast CT is fastest, most sensitive, and most specific modality to demonstrate subarachnoid hemorrhage
- More sensitive than MRI for detection of calcifications (lesions that have a strong tendency to calcify are caused by toxoplasmosis, craniopharyngioma, chondrosarcoma, retinoblastoma, tuberous clerosis, and Sturge-Weber syndrome)
- Preferred to MRI in facial or head trauma, postoperative craniotomy, and sinusitis patients
- Inflammatory or congenital lesions of the temporal bone also better visualized with CT than MRI

Weaknesses

- Less sensitive to parenchymal lesions and leptomeningeal processes, particularly white matter lesions, than MRI
- Potential for significant contrast reaction
- Not useful for evaluation of tissue perfusion, metabolism, or vessel blood flow

Comments

- Noncontrast CT of the brain is often used as the initial imaging modality for patients suspected of having had a stroke (Fig. 1-40) and in patients with suspected subarachnoid hemorrhage (SAH) (Fig. 1-41).
- Enhanced images are indicated when infection, inflammation or neoplasia, and seizures are suspected.
- Unenhanced images are indicated in hemorrhagic or ischemic events, head trauma, congenital anomalies, and degenerative diseases.
- On CT of the brain, hemorrhage will be denser than surrounding brain tissue but not as dense as calcium or bone.
- Patients with acute infarcts often have a "normal" CT scan initially. Early findings will be due to edema in the affected portion of the brain. Subacute findings include an increase in the mass effect. A wedge-shaped hypodense area extending to the cortex or involving the basal ganglia, thalamus, or brainstem will develop.
- In *subdural hematoma*, CT reveals a concave blood collection between skull and brain. It will cross suture lines but will not cross the midline. Contrast-enhanced CT will accentuate the nonenhancing subdural blood.
- In *epidural hematoma,* CT reveals a biconvex hyperdense blood collection with significant mass effect and brain edema. It will not cross suture lines.
- In cases where the detection of calcium is important, noncontrast CT is preferred.
- New Orleans Criteria recommend CT after minor head injury if the patient meets one or more of the following criteria: headache, vomiting, age older than 60 years, drug or alcohol intoxication, persistent anterograde amnesia (deficits in short-term memory), visible trauma above clavicle, or seizure.

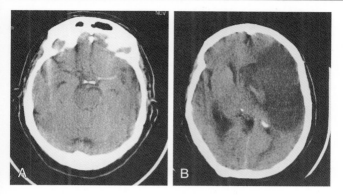

Figure 1-40 A, Axial, noncontrast CT demonstrates a dense left middle cerebral artery, indicating thrombus in the horizontal segment of the left middle cerebral artery. **B,** Scan performed 24 hours after the initial study demonstrates a large acute infarct in the distribution of the left middle cerebral artery (MCA) with mass effect and midline shift.   *(From Specht N: Practical Guide to Diagnostic Imaging, St. Louis, Mosby, 1998.)*

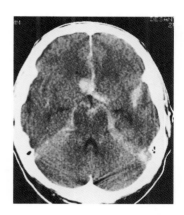

Figure 1-41 Noncontrast CT demonstrates diffuse subarachnoid hemorrhage. The rounded area of hyperdensity anterior to the suprasellar cistern represents an aneurysm of the anterior communicating artery.   *(From Specht N: Practical Guide to Diagnostic Imaging, St. Louis, Mosby, 1998.)*

- Cost: CT of head without contrast $$; CT of head with contrast $$$; CT of head with and without contrast $$$

2. MRI of Brain

Indications
- Suspected brain neoplasm (primary or metastatic)
- Suspected demyelinating diseases of brain (e.g., multiple sclerosis)
- Suspected sellar and parasellar abnormalities
- Suspected brain abscess and cerebritis
- Suspected granulomatous, fungal, and parasitic encephalopathies
- Suspected encephalitis (much more sensitive than CT)

- Suspected congenital malformations (e.g., Chiari malformations, corpus callosum abnormalities, cephaloceles)
- Stroke evaluation (more sensitive than CT)
- After trauma to evaluate for diffuse axonal injury

Strengths
- Noninvasive
- Generally safe contrast agent
- No ionizing radiation
- Soft tissue resolution
- Multiplanar

Weaknesses
- Expensive
- Needs cooperative patient
- Time consuming
- Not as sensitive as CT for detection of subarachnoid hemorrhage
- Insensitive to the presence of calcification and bone
- CT preferred to MRI in facial or head trauma, postoperative craniotomy, and sinusitis patients
- Inflammatory or congenital lesions of temporal bone also better visualized with CT than MRI
- Cannot be performed in patients with non–MR-compatible aneurysm clips pacemaker, cochlear implants, or metallic foreign body in eyes; safe in women with IUDs (including copper ones), and those with surgical clips and staples

Comments
- MRI is the imaging procedure of choice for evaluation of suspected brain tumor, intracranial mass, suspected pituitary and juxtasellar lesions, cerebellar and

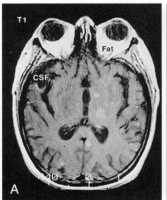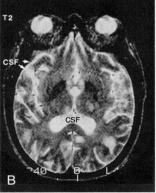

Figure 1-42 MR images of the brain. A wide variety of imaging parameters can make tissues appear different. The two most common presentations are T1-weighted images (**A**) in which fat appears white, water and cerebrospinal fluid appear black, and brain and muscle appear gray. In almost all MR images, bone gives off no signal and appears black. **B,** With T2-weighted imaging, fat is dark and water and cerebrospinal fluid have a high signal and appear bright or white. The brain and soft tissues still appear gray. (*From Mettler FA: Primary Care Radiology. Philadelphia, WB Saunders, 2000.*)

brainstem symptoms, hydrocephalus, lesions of visual system, congenital CNS abnormalities, and suspected structural abnormalities related to epilepsy.

- MRI is superior to CT in the initial diagnosis of acute stroke. Most of the superiority of MRI is attributed to its ability to detect acute ischemic stroke. It is now rapidly available in many centers and preferred by most physicians as the initial imaging modality in patients with suspected acute stroke.
- Enhanced images are indicated when infection, inflammation, neoplasia, and seizures are suspected. Contrast may also be required in evaluation of demyelinating disorders to identify small plaques in the region of optic nerves.
- Unenhanced images are indicated in hemorrhagic or ischemic events, head trauma, congenital anomalies, and degenerative diseases.
- Figs. 1-42 and 1-43 describe imaging parameters and normal anatomy of the brain on MRI. When white matter disease (e.g., MS) is suspected, the

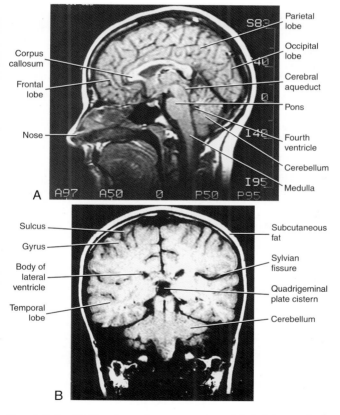

Figure 1-43 **A** and **B**, Normal magnetic resonance anatomy of the brain in coronal and sagittal projections. *(From Mettler FA: Primary Care Radiology, Philadelphia, WB Saunders, 2000.)*

best imaging test is MRI with fluid attenuated inversion recovery (FLAIR) images.

- When subarachnoid hemorrhage is suspected, MRI is not preferred as the initial study. Noncontrast CT is the fastest, most sensitive, and most specific modality to demonstrate subarachnoid hemorrhage.
- Dedicated protocols can evaluate the orbits, sella, and cerebellopontine angles with thin cuts and superior detail to CT.
- Anxious patients (especially those with claustrophobia) should be premedicated with an anxiolytic agent, and their imaging should be done with "open MRI" whenever possible.
- Cost: MRI of brain without contrast $$$$; MRI of brain with contrast $$$$; MRI of brain with and without contrast $$$$$

I. Positron Emission Tomography (PET)

Indications

- Diagnosis, staging, and restaging of lung cancer (non–small cell), esophageal cancer, colorectal cancer, head and neck cancer (excluding CNS and thyroid), lymphoma (Fig. 1-44), melanoma
- Breast cancer: as an adjunct to standard imaging modalities in staging (patients with distant metastasis) and restaging (patients with local/regional recurrence or metastasis)
- Breast cancer: as an adjunct to standard imaging modalities for monitoring tumor response to treatment for women with locally advanced and metastatic breast cancer when a change in therapy is anticipated
- Presurgical evaluation for refractory seizures
- Evaluation for myocardial viability prior to revascularization
- Evaluation for the presence of malignancy in a pulmonary nodule
- Evaluation of Alzheimer's disease and frontal lobe dementias

Strengths

- Can detect malignant involvement of small nodes (unlike CT, which looks for lymph node enlargement to detect malignancy)
- Can detect malignancy in tumor sites that have same appearance as adjacent normal structures on CT
- Useful in detecting unknown sites of metastatic disease and reducing futile thoracotomies in patients with non–small cell lung cancer
- Useful in evaluation of pulmonary nodules (a nodule that demonstrates F-18 fluorodeoxyglucose [FDG] uptake on PET typically warrants biopsy)
- Useful to differentiate residual masses due to scar tissue versus active lymphoma in post–lymphoma therapy patients
- Useful to identify Alzheimer's disease and frontal lobe dementias (e.g., Pick's disease)

Weaknesses

- Poor visualization of neoplasms that are not very metabolically active or are unable to retain FDG (e.g., hepatocellular carcinoma, prostate cancer, bronchoalveolar lung cancer)
- Decreased sensitivity in patients with diabetes
- Poor imaging of brain metastases due to an overall significant amount of increased FDG uptake in the brain (high background activity)
- Poor visualization of very small lung metastases (<5 mm)

FDG-PET at diagnosis

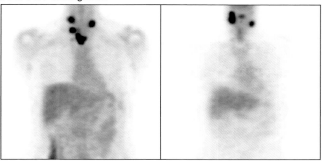

FDG-PET 2 months later after 3 cycles of R-CHOP

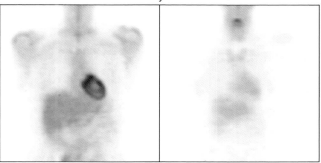

Figure 1-44 FDG-PET scan before and after treatment with rituximab, cyclophosphamide, doxorubicin, Oncovin, and prednisolone (R-CHOP). Resolution of cervical and upper mediastinal disease is shown. *(From Young NS, Gerson SL, High KA, eds: Clinical Hematology, St. Louis, Mosby, 2006.)*

- Unable to distinguish malignancy from inflammatory disease (e.g., sarcoidosis, TB) due to increased FDG uptake by active granulomatous disease
- Not useful in defining regional draining lymph nodes in melanoma (sentinel node biopsy is superior)
- Expensive
- Limited availability

Comments

- PET captures chemical and physiologic changes related to metabolism, as opposed to gross anatomy and structure. Many types of neoplasms demonstrate an increased uptake of glucose. A PET camera measures radiolabeled phosphorylated FDG to determine increased cellular activity typical of many types of neoplasms.

- Rubidium-82, a tracer used for PET myocardial perfusion imaging, localizes in the myocardium in proportion to regional blood flow. It can be used to evaluate myocardial viability to accurately predict which patients will have significant improvement in left ventricular function after revascularization.
- PET imaging in early Alzheimer's disease reveals decreased metabolic activity in the mesial temporal, posterior temporal, and parietal lobes. This is useful to distinguish Alzheimer's dementia from Pick's disease and other frontal lobe dementias (decreased metabolic activity in frontal lobes)
- Costs associated with PET scanning and its availability are major limiting factors to its use.
- Cost: $$$$ for PET of body, extremity, abdomen, brain metabolic, brain perfusion; $$$$ for cardiac PET

J. Single-Photon Emission Computed Tomography

Indications
- Evaluation of coronary artery disease
- Evaluation of CNS diseases, including epilepsy, cerebrovascular disease, and psychiatric disorders
- Can help provide three-dimensional evaluation of lesions in bone scanning, hepatobiliary imaging, and other areas of nuclear medicine

Strengths
- Contrast resolution higher than with planar images
- Useful for epilepsy and coronary artery disease
- Easier to implement than PET
- Improved sensitivity of diagnosis of coronary disease and delineation of the size of ischemic or infarcted myocardium
- Regional cerebral blood flow (CBF) brain SPECT useful to identify patients at risk for stroke who may benefit from neurosurgical revascularization procedures
- Tracer iodine-123 IBZM can map the dopamine D2 receptor and is useful in evaluation of movement disorders and schizophrenia
- Cerebral necrosis following brain tumor therapy cannot be distinguished from residual or recurrent tumor by either CT or MRI; SPECT useful to distinguish between new or residual glioblastoma (Fig. 1-45) following surgery and brain necrosis

Weaknesses
- Resolution not as good as MRI/CT
- Expensive
- Not readily available

Comments
- SPECT is a technique that uses one, two, or three gamma cameras to record activity emitted from multiple projections around the patient.
- Brain SPECT applications use the radionuclide Tc-99m HMPAO, a brain flow tracer that is extracted by the brain in proportion to regional cerebral blood flow.
- Cost: $$$

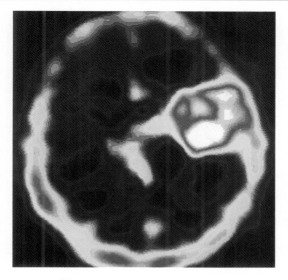

Figure 1-45 ²⁰¹T1 SPECT in a 40-year-old man with a left frontotemporal mass on MRI. High uptake typical of high-grade glioma, which was confirmed on biopsy to be a glioblastoma. *(Image courtesy of Professor Donald M. Hadley, Glasgow. From Grainger RG, Allison D: Grainger & Allison's Diagnostic Radiology: A Textbook of Medical Imaging, Churchill Livingstone, ed 4, 2001.)*

K.   Vascular Imaging

1. Angiography

Indications
- Cerebral angiography: evaluation for vascular lesions of the brain (Fig. 1-46) and great vessels of the neck (aneurysm, arteriovenous malformation [AVM], vasculitis)
- Thoracic aorta: chest trauma, suspected dissection, aneurysm, evaluation of vascular anatomy and anomaly, aortic mass (neoplasm, non-neoplastic), vasculitis
- Abdominal aorta: abdominal trauma, aneurysm, vasculitis, preoperative evaluation, peripheral vascular disease
- Renal: renal artery stenosis, renovascular hypertension, trauma, renal vein thrombosis, vasculitis, neoplasm, transplanar, AVM
- Mesenteric: GI hemorrhage, AVM, angiodysplasia, intestinal ischemia, splenic/splanchnic aneurysm, neoplasm
- Hepatic: neoplasm, pretransplant assessment, AVM, focal nodular hyperplasia

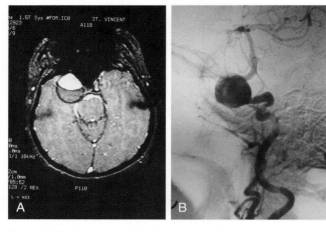

Figure 1-46 Cerebral aneurysm. **A**, Axial, noncontrast gradient-echo image demonstrates a giant aneurysm in the medial portion of the right middle cranial fossa. The area of increased signal intensity represents the lumen of the aneurysm. **B**, Right carotid arteriogram (oblique view of the same patient) demonstrates a giant aneurysm of the distal right internal carotid artery. *(From Specht N: Practical Guide to Diagnostic Imaging, St. Louis, Mosby, 1998.)*

- Subclavian: aneurysm, AVM, arterial insufficiency, trauma
- Splenic: trauma, neoplasm, aneurysm
- Pancreatic: evaluation and staging of neoplasm, localization of islet cell tumor
- Bronchial: refractory hemoptysis, AVM, pulmonary sequestration
- Pulmonary: PE, vaculitis, AVM, congenital vascular lesions
- Cardiac: evaluation of coronary anatomy; severity of valvular disease; diseases of the myocardium, pericardium, or endocardium; congenital defects; pulmonary hypertension; therapeutic procedures (angioplasty, embolization, selective drug therapy)
- Detection of superior sagittal sinus thrombosis
- Pre–transphenoidal hypophysectomy assessment

Strengths
- Most accurate method for evaluation of vasculature
- Best modality for preoperative assessment and delineation of branch vessel involvement
- Allows intervention (e.g., percutaneous transluminal angioplasty [PTA], renal artery angioplasty, intravascular stents, delivery of therapeutic agents, thrombolysis, embolization of aneurysms or intrabdominal/pelvic bleeding)

Weaknesses
- Invasive
- Low but significant risk of mortality (<0.05%) and morbidity (e.g., local complications at catheter insertion area, contrast reaction, renal insufficiency, thrombosis, embolism)

- Expensive
- Poor visualization of mural thrombus or extravascular hematoma
- Does not provide information about the disease process that takes place in the vessel wall

Comments
- Angiography is the gold standard for evaluation of vascular lesions and aortic dissection.
- Relative contraindications are coagulopathy, renal insufficiency, allergy to contrast agents, uncontrolled CHF, and metformin use within 48 hours.
- Cost: $$$$

2. Aorta Ultrasound

Indications
- Suspected aneurysm (Fig. 1-47)
- Arterial dissection

Strengths
- Fast
- Noninvasive
- No radiation
- Can be performed at bedside
- Can be repeated serially

Weaknesses
- Operator dependent; results may be affected by skill of technician
- Retained barium from x-ray procedures will interfere with interpretation

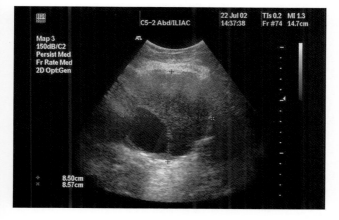

Figure 1-47 Ultrasound appearance of an abdominal aortic aneurysm (AAA), seen in cross-section. Sonography is highly accurate in diagnosing and measuring infrarenal aortic aneurysms. *(Courtesy M. Ellis. From Crawford, MH, DiMarco JP, Paulus WJ, eds: Cardiology, ed 2, St. Louis, Mosby, 2004.)*

Comments
• Ultrasound is ideal for following aneurysm progression over time.
• Cost: $$

3. Arterial Ultrasound

Indications
• Suspected aneurysm
• Arterial dissection
• Arterial stenosis
• Arterial occlusion
• Suspected AV fistula or pseudoaneurysm
• Image guidance for thrombin injection of pseudoaneurysm

Strengths
• Fast
• Noninvasive
• No radiation
• Can be performed at bedside
• Can be repeated serially

Weaknesses
• Operator dependent; results may be affected by skill of technician
• Retained barium from x-ray procedures will interfere with interpretation

Comments
• Ultrasound is ideal for following aneurysm progression over time.
• Useful as a screening method for suspected AV fistula.
• Doppler ultrasound can be used to study the patency of grafts because it can provide a measurement of flow volume/unit time.
• Cost: $$

4. Captopril Renal Scan (CRS)

Indications
• Detection of renal artery stenosis in the setting of clinically suspected renovascular hypertension
• Evaluation for revascularization in patient with known renal artery stenosis

Strengths
• Noninvasive

Weaknesses
• Limited use as screening method for renal artery stenosis due to low specificity and sensitivity
• Drop in systemic blood pressure following administration of angiotensin-converting enzyme (ACE) inhibitors may interfere with test interpretation
• Poor renal function from any cause makes interpretation difficult

Comments
• CRS involves two radionuclide studies, one with and one without captopril. In patients with hemodynamically significant renal artery stenosis, delayed uptake and cortical retention in the affected kidney will occur (Fig. 1-48).
• Because a change in the glomerular filtration rate (GFR) on renal scan after administration of captopril suggests that renal artery stenosis is more likely to be hemodynamically significant, the appropriate use of CRS should be in

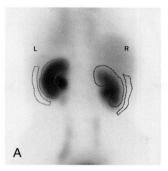

Captopril-enhanced renography

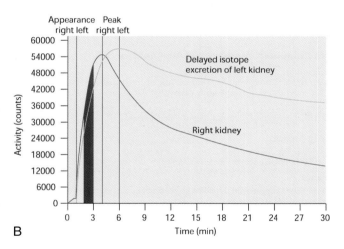

Figure 1-48 Captopril-enhanced renography. **A**, Scan in a patient with newly developing hypertension. **B**, Renogram demonstrates delayed arrival and excretion of isotope (MAG3) in the affected left kidney.   *(From Johnson RJ, Feehally J: Comprehensive Clinical Nephrology, ed 2, St. Louis, Mosby, 2000.)*

patients with known renal artery stenosis (by renal arteriography or MRA) who are considered for revascularization.
• Cost: $$

5. Carotid Ultrasonography

Indications
• Screening for extracranial vascular disease primarily at the carotid bifurcation

Strengths
- Noninvasive
- Safe
- No ionizing radiation

Weaknesses
- Operator dependent; can be significantly influenced by skills and bias of operator
- Of limited utility for disease above the region of the carotid bifurcation
- In 10% of patients, carotid bifurcation lies above angle of jaw, making ultrasound difficult or impossible
- Subject to errors of interpretation in cases of high-grade stenoses or complete occlusion
- Calcified plaques interfere with visualization of vascular lumen
- Difficulty visualizing tandem lesions
- Echolucency of acute thrombi (indistinguishable from flowing blood)

Comments
- Carotid arteriography is necessary when surgical intervention is contemplated.
- Duplex color flow Doppler is the best initial screening test to evaluate the carotid arteries.
- Cost: $$

6. Computed Tomographic Angiography (CTA)

Indications
- Screening of asymptomatic patients at risk for cerebral aneurysms
- Rapid evaluation of symptomatic patients for aneurysms

Strengths
- Artifact is less than with conventional angiography
- Fast
- High sensitivity
- Noninvasive
- Not affected by flow-related effects seen with MRA
- Does not involve MRI compatibility problems (e.g., pacemakers, metallic clips)
- Can detect intraluminal thrombus, calcification in the neck of an aneurysm, and extravascular hematoma
- Can reveal complications of aneurysms (e.g., compression of other structures, bone erosion)

Weaknesses
- Use of ionizing radiation
- Injection of IV iodine (potential for contrast reaction)
- Excessive length of time for processing of data after test
- Poor visualization of vessels at base of skull
- May produce artifacts due to calcifications in walls of vessels and aneurysm clips
- Cannot be repeated (unlike MRA)
- Does not reliably delineate involvement of branch vessels
- Poor visualization of entry and re-entry sites when evaluating aortic dissection

Comments
- In CTA, IV contrast and a thin-slice helical CT are used to create a three-dimensional view of blood vessels.
- CTA is an alternative to MRA for evaluation of extracranial and intracranial vasculature.
- Cost: $$$

7. Magnetic Resonance Angiography (MRA)

Indications

- Evaluation of extracranial vasculature for the presence of lesions of the carotid artery, extracranial vasculitis (e.g., giant cell arteritis), congenital vascular abnormalities (e.g., fibromuscular disease), dissection of vertebral and carotid arteries, and extracranial traumatic fistula.
- Suspected intracranial aneurysm
- Follow-up of unruptured intracranial aneurysm
- Follow-up of treated aneurysm when conventional angiography is contraindicated
- Workup of intracranial vasculitis
- Intracranial venous occlusive disease
- Intracranial vascular compression syndromes
- Definition of blood supply to vascular neoplasms
- Evaluation of AVMs

Strengths

- Noninvasive and readily repeatable
- Safe, no ionizing radiation
- Useful screening tool for both extracranial and intracranial vascular disease (Fig. 1-49)

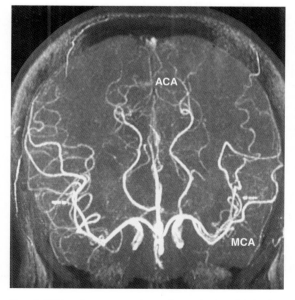

Figure 1-49 Magnetic resonance angiogram. An anterior view of the head shows intracerebral vessels, including the anterior cerebral artery (ACA) and the middle cerebral artery (MCA). These images were obtained without injection of any contrast agent. (*From Mettler FA: Primary Care Radiology, Philadelphia, WB Saunders, 2000.*)

- May be performed without contrast
- Images can be reconstructed in any plane
- Can be used safely in patients with renal insufficiency
- Unlike CTA or conventional angiography, able to demonstrate both anatomy and flow rate
- In severe (70%-99%) carotid stenosis, is 95% sensitive and 90% specific versus 86% sensitivity and 87% specificity for duplex ultrasonography

Weaknesses
- Requires cooperative patient
- Need contrast to image distal vessels adequately
- May overestimate degree of vascular stenosis
- May miss small aneurysms (<3 mm)
- Use instead of conventional angiography may preclude other diagnoses; for example, in patients with suspected carotid stenosis, additional vascular lesions such as brain AVM will be missed if only extracranial MRA is performed
- Cannot be performed in patients with non–MR-compatible aneurysm clips, pacemaker, cochlear implants, or metallic foreign body in eyes; safe in women with IUDs (including copper ones), and those with surgical clips and staples
- Poor visualization of ulcerations in atheromas
- Images of distal intracranial vessels generally difficult to interpret
- Slow blood flow in a vessel with high-grade stenosis may be falsely interpreted as occlusion (has surgical implications because surgery is often performed for stenosis and not for vascular occlusion)
- Sensitivity to motion (e.g., ventilation) limits use in thoracic region
- Peristaltic motion in abdomen may interfere with interpretation

Comments
- Although conventional angiography remains the definitive diagnostic modality for evaluation of intracranial aneurysm, MRA is rapidly replacing it for initial evaluation of cerebral vasculature.
- MRI contrast agents (when used) are less allergenic and nephrotoxic than conventional iodinated contrast agents.
- Anxious patients (especially those with claustrophobia) should be premedicated with an anxiolitic agent, and their imaging should be done with "open MRI" whenever possible.
- Cost: MRA without contrast $$$$

8. Magnetic Resonance Direct Thrombus Imaging (MRDTI)

Indication
- Diagnosis of deep vein thrombosis (DVT)

Strengths
- Noninvasive
- Highly reproducible interpretation
- Accurate in diagnosing isolated calf and proximal DVT
- Useful to determine thrombus age
- Does not require contrast or special patient preparation
- Can be performed in patient with full length leg plaster cast
- Can be repeated serially to monitor thrombus progression
- Safe in pregnancy

Weaknesses
- High cost
- Not readily available
- Needs cooperative patient
- Time consuming
- Cannot be performed in patients with non–MR-compatible aneurysm clips, pacemaker, cochlear implants, or metallic foreign body in eyes; safe in women with IUDs (including copper ones), and those with surgical clips and staples

Comments
- MRDTI is useful and well tolerated in pregnancy, in patients with full leg plaster casts, and in patients with isolated calf DVT (present in 5% of patients with suspected DVT).
- This is a reliable test for asymptomatic thrombosis because it does not depend on the filling of the lumen or distribution of blood flow and can image small-volume thrombi.
- Anxious patients (especially those with claustrophobia) should be premedicated with an anxiolitic agent, and their imaging should be done with "open MRI" whenever possible.
- Cost: $$$$

9. Pulmonary Angiography

Indications
- Diagnosis of pulmonary embolism in patients with inconclusive ventilation/perfusion (V/Q) scan (Fig. 1-50)
- Vasculitis
- AVM
- Congenital vascular lesion

Strengths
- Sensitivity 98%, specificity 97% for PE
- Allows simultaneous adjunctive procedures (e.g., placement of inferior vena cava (IVC) filter, thrombectomy, local catheter-directed thrombectomy)

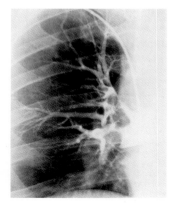

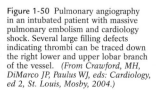

Figure 1-50 Pulmonary angiography in an intubated patient with massive pulmonary embolism and cardiology shock. Several large filling defects indicating thrombi can be traced down the right lower and upper lobar branch of the vessel. *(From Crawford, MH, DiMarco JP, Paulus WJ, eds: Cardiology, ed 2, St. Louis, Mosby, 2004.)*

Weaknesses
- Requires IV contrast (potential for significant contrast reaction)
- Invasive
- Expensive

Comments
- Pulmonary angiography is the gold standard test for PE.
- Improvement in CT technology has diminished the use of pulmonary angiography for evaluation of PE.
- This test is generally used as a second-line diagnostic test in patients with an indeterminate V/Q scan.
- Relative contraindications are coagulopathy, renal insufficiency, allergy to contrast agents, uncontrolled CHF, and metformin use within 48 hours.
- LBBB and increased pulmonary artery pressure are contraindications to pulmonary angiography.
- Cost: $$$$

10. Transcranial Doppler

Indications
- Evaluation of the basal cerebral arteries
- Detection of cerebrovascular spasm (e.g., after surgery, after subarachnoid hemorrhage)
- Evaluation of middle cerebral artery patency in patients with carotid stenosis

Strengths
- Noninvasive
- Can provide indirect information about extracranial arterial occlusive disease and can evaluate the intracranial carotids and the circle of Willis
- No ionizing radiation
- Fast

Weaknesses
- Operator dependent; can be significantly influenced by the skills and bias of the operator

Comments
- Transcranial Doppler uses low-frequency ultrasonography to evaluate the flow velocity spectrum of the cerebral vessels.
- Cost: $$

11. Venography

Indications
- Suspected DVT
- Performed prior to IVC filter placement

Strengths
- Most reliable test for diagnosis of asymptomatic thrombus and thrombus isolated within calf or pelvis

Weaknesses
- Potential for significant contrast reactions
- Invasive
- Inadequate imaging in the pelvis
- Insufficient delineation of the proximal extent of thrombosis in patients with above-knee DVT
- High interobserver variability (>10%)

Comments
- Venography is the gold standard for diagnosis of DVT.
- It is generally used only when other tests for DVT are inconclusive and clinical suspicion is high.
- Cost: $$

12. Venous Doppler Ultrasound

Indications
- Suspected DVT (Fig. 1-51)
- Follow-up exam to evaluate propagation of venous thrombus
- Source evaluation for known or suspected PE
- Chronic venous insufficiency
- Swollen and/or painful leg

Strengths
- Noninvasive
- Fast
- Can be repeated serially
- Readily available
- Inexpensive

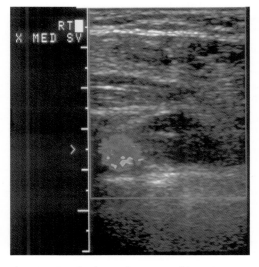

Figure 1-51 Doppler ultrasound appearance of deep vein thrombosis. The superficial femoral vein is filled with echogenic material representing thrombus, and no flow can be identified in the vein on Doppler evaluation. Flow can be identified in the adjacent artery on color Doppler evaluations *(arrows)*. *(From Crawford, MH, DiMarco JP, Paulus WJ, eds: Cardiology, ed 2, St. Louis, Mosby, 2004.)*

- Can be performed at bedside
- No ionizing radiation

Weaknesses
- Poor visualization of pelvic and calf veins
- Negative test does not conclusively "rule out" DVT at presentation; repeat examination after 5 to 7 days may be necessary to exclude clinically suspected thrombosis in symptomatic patients
- Operator dependent; results may be affected by skill of technician

Comments
- Venous Doppler is the initial test of choice in suspected DVT.
- Cost: $

13. Ventilation/Perfusion Lung Scan (V/Q SCAN)

Indications
- Suspected PE
- Suspected right-to-left shunt
- Evaluation of relative lung function before surgery (quantitative V/Q scan)

Strengths
- Noninvasive
- Widely available
- High sensitivity (>95%)

Weaknesses
- Low specificity
- Cannot be used in patients with baseline chest film abnormalities
- Cannot differentiate acute from chronic PE
- More than 70% of scans nondiagnostic
- Results can be equivocal in patients with preexisting lung disease

Comments
- A "matched defect" (area not ventilated and not perfused) can occur with COPD, tumors, lung infarction, airspace disease, asthma.
- A "V/Q mismatch" (area ventilated but not perfused) occurs with PE, vasculitis, radiation therapy, tumor compressing the pulmonary artery, and fibrosing mediastinitis compressing the pulmonary artery.
- A "reverse mismatched defect" (area perfused but not ventilated) can occur with mucus plugging, pneumonia, and alveolar pulmonary edema.
- A "normal" V/Q scan has a high predictive value for PE (<5% probability)
- A "high-probability" V/Q scan (two or more large mismatched segmental defects or any combination of mismatched defects equivalent to two large segmental defects; Fig. 1-52) has a high positive predictive value (>85% for PE).
- A nondiagnostic "intermediate" VQ scan should be interpreted in the context of clinical suspicion and additional testing (e.g., D-dimer test).
- Patient must be cooperative enough to perform the ventilation portion of the examination. If defects are seen on the perfusion study and the patient cannot tolerate or perform the ventilation portion, the examination is then indeterminate and further evaluation is necessary.
- CT is an excellent alternative to V/Q because CT can provide more information, is more specific, and can provide alternate reasons for patients' dyspnea or chest pain. Computed tomographic pulmonary angiography (CTPA) has in many centers replaced ventilation/perfusion lung scanning because it provides a clear result (either positive or negative) and because it may detect alternative nonthrombotic causes of patients' symptoms.
- Cost: $$$

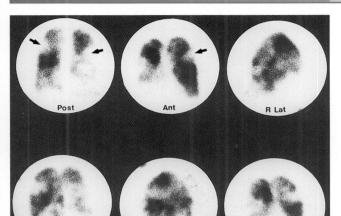

Figure 1-52 Multiple pulmonary emboli. This young lady with shortness of breath had a normal chest radiograph and a normal ventilation lung scan. The images here are from the perfusion portion of the nuclear medicine lung scan. Note the multiple segmental and subsegmental areas without perfusion *(arrows)* throughout both lungs. This is indicative of a high probability of pulmonary emboli. *Post,* posterior; *Ant,* anterior; *R Lat,* right lateral; *LPO,* left posterior oblique; *L Lat,* left lateral; *RAO,* right anterior oblique. *(From Mettler FA: Primary Care Radiology, Philadelphia, WB Saunders, 2000.)*

L. Oncology

1. Whole-body Integrated (Dual-modality) Positron Emission Tomography (PET) and CT (PET-CT)

Indications
- Identification and determination of the extent of malignant disease and monitoring therapy of numerous cancers (Fig. 1-53)
- Workup of solitary pulmonary nodules
- Staging of lung cancer
- Evaluation of carcinoma of unknown primary origin
- Restaging cancer; valuable in two groups of patients: those in whom other imaging or laboratory studies raise the concern of relapse, and those in whom the response to treatment needs to be evaluated
- Evaluation of efficacy of cancer chemotherapy
- Medicare-accepted indications for PET scanning include: diagnosis, staging, and restaging of lymphoma, melanoma, lung cancer, head and neck cancer, and esophageal cancer; also includes staging, restaging, and evaluating treatment response to breast cancer and restaging of thyroid cancer (with negative iodine-131 scan and positive thyroglobulin)

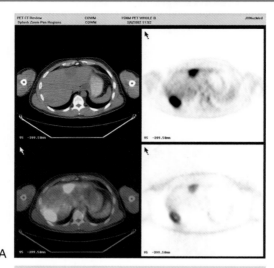

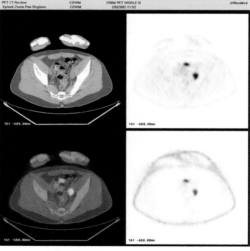

Figure 1-53 Colon cancer. **A,** PET and CT image display of a patient with two FDG-avid lesions in the liver. These are seen on the CT *(upper left)* scan, attenuation-corrected PET *(upper right)* scan, non–attenuation-corrected PET *(lower right)* scan, and fused images *(lower left).* **B,** PET and CT images of the pelvis, oriented as in **A,** show increased FDG uptake in a left external iliac lymph node metastasis. *(From Abeloff MD: Clinical Oncology, ed 3, Philadelphia, 2004, Elsevier.)*

Strengths
- Noninvasive
- In addition to its application in oncology, also useful in cardiology to detect coronary artery disease and to assess whether dysfunctional myocardial tissue is viable, and in neurology and psychiatry in differentiating between tumor recurrence and radiation necrosis, differentiating Alzheimer's disease from other dementias, and locating epileptic foci

Weaknesses
- Less sensitive in detecting small neoplasms due to limited spatial resolution

Comments
- The effective radiation dose from a single PET scan is relatively small (10 mSv). The effective dose for PET-CT is 20 mSv because a whole-body CT is performed in conjunction with PET. However, even when more than one PET-CT scan is performed during follow-up of patients with certain types of cancer after therapy, the cumulative effective dose is similar to that of the same number of "dedicated" contrast-enhanced CT scans which are often performed during follow-up.
- Cost: $$$$

2. Whole-Body MRI

Indications
- Detection of skeletal metastases as an alternative to skeletal scintigraphy
- Evaluation of total tumor burden, particularly in patients whose tumors spread preferentially to brain, bone, and liver, such as breast and lung tumors

Strengths
- Better detection of lesions in the spine and pelvis than scintigraphy
- Noninvasive
- Safe contrast agent (MRI uses gadolinium, an IV agent that is less nephrotoxic)
- No ionizing radiation
- Soft-tissue resolution
- Multiplanar

Weaknesses
- Expensive
- Needs cooperative patient
- Time consuming
- Cannot be performed in patients with non–MR compatible aneurysm clips, pacemaker, cochlear implants, or metallic foreign body in eyes; safe in women with IUDs (including copper ones), and those with surgical clips and staples

Comments
- Nononcologic applications of whole-body MRI include: identifying sites suitable for percutaneous biopsy, particularly in immunocompromised hosts, evaluation of whole-body fat measurements and body composition research, evaluation of suspected polymyositis.
- Anxious patients (especially those with claustrophobia) should be premedicated with an anxiolytic agent, and their imaging should be done with "open MRI" whenever possible.
- Cost: $$$$

REFERENCES

1. Ali A, Santini JM, Vardo J: Video capsule endoscopy: a voyage beyond the end of the scope, *Cleveland Clinic J* 71:415-424, 2004.
2. American Heart Association: AHA guidelines on cardiac CT for assessing coronary artery disease, *Circulation*, October 17, 2006.
3. Anderson DR et al: Computed tomographic pulmonary angiography vs ventilation-perfusion lung scanning in patients with suspected pulmonary embolism, *JAMA* 298(23):2743-2753, 2007.
4. Carman TL, Deitcher SR: Advances in diagnosing and excluding pulmonary embolism: spiral CT and D-Dimer measurement, *Cleveland Clinic J Med* 69:721-728, 2002.
5. Chalia JA et al: Magnetic resonance imaging and computed tomography in emergency assessment of patients with suspected acute stroke: a prospective comparison, *Lancet* 369: 293-298, 2007.
6. Colli A et al: Accuracy of ultrasonography, spiral CT, magnetic resonance, and alpha-fetoprotein in diagnosing hepatocellular carcinoma: a systematic review, *Am J Gastroenterol* 101:513-523, 2006.
7. Dumot JA: ERCP: current uses and less-invasive options, *Cleveland Clinic J Med* 73:418-441, 2006.
8. Ebell MH: Computed tomography after minor head injury, *Am Fam Physician* 73:2205-2206, 2006.
9. Fenton JJ, Taplin SH et al: Influence of computer-aided detection on performance of screening mammography, *N Eng J Med* 356:1399-1409, 2007.
10. Fraser DGW et al: Diagnosis of lower-limb deep venous thrombosis: a prospective blinded study of Magnetic Resonance Direct Thrombus Imaging, *Ann Intern Med* 135:89-98, 2002.
11. Gay SB, Woodcock RJ: *Radiology recall*, Philadelphia, Lippincott Williams & Wilkins, 2000.
12. Goldman L, Bennet JC, eds: *Cecil textbook of medicine*, ed 21, Philadelphia, WB Saunders 2000.
13. Hassan C et al: Computed tomographic colonography to screen for colorectal cancer, extracolonic cancer, and aortic aneurysm, *Arch Intern Med* 168(7):696-706, 2008.
14. Huot SJ et al: Utility of captopril renal scans for detecting renal artery stenosis, *Arch Intern Med* 162:1981-1984, 2002.
15. Juweid ME, Cheson BD: Positron-emission tomography and assessment of cancer therapy, *N Engl J Med* 354:496-507, 2006.
16. Kim DH et al: CT colonography versus colonoscopy for the detection of advanced neoplasia, *N Engl J Med*: 357:1403-1412, 2007.
17. Lehman CD et al: MRI evaluation of the contralateral breast in women with recently diagnosed breast cancer, *N Engl J Med* 356:1295-1303, 2003.
18. Mettler FA: *Primary care radiology*, Philadelphia, WB Saunders 2000.
19. Noto RB: Positron emission tomography: the basics, *R I Med J* 86:29-132, 2003.
20. Orrison WW et al: *Pocket medical imaging consultant*, Houston, Healthhelp, 2002.
21. Romagnuolo J et al: Magnetic resonance cholangiopancreatography: a meta-analysis of test performance in suspected biliary disease, *Ann Intern Med* 139:547-557, 2003.
22. Specht NT, Russo RD: *Practical guide to diagnostic imaging*, St. Louis, Mosby, 1998.
23. Stein PD et al: Multidetector computed tomography for the diagnosis of coronary artery disease: a systematic review, *Am J Med* 119:203-216, 2006.
24. Thrall JH, Ziessman HA: *Nuclear medicine: the requisites,* St. Louis, Mosby, 1995.
25. Weissleder R, Wittenberg J, Harisinghani MG, Chen JW: *Primer of diagnostic imaging*, ed 4, St. Louis, Mosby, 2007.

Laboratory Values
and Interpretation of Results

This section covers 313 laboratory tests. Each test is approached with the following format:
- Laboratory test
- Normal range in adult patients
- Common abnormalities (e.g., positive test, increased or decreased value)
- Causes of abnormal result

The normal ranges may differ slightly, depending on the laboratory. The reader should be aware of the "normal range" of the particular laboratory performing the test. Every attempt has been made to present current laboratory test data with emphasis on practical considerations. It's important to remember that lab tests do not make diagnoses, doctors do. As such any lab results should be integrated with the complete clinical picture and radiographic studies (if needed) to make a diagnosis.

ACE LEVEL; SEE ANGIOTENSIN-CONVERTING ENZYME
ACETONE (SERUM OR PLASMA)

Normal: negative

Elevated in: diabetic ketoacidosis (DKA), starvation, isopropanol ingestion

ACETYLCHOLINE RECEPTOR (AChR) ANTIBODY

Normal: < 0.03 nmol/L

Elevated in: myasthenia gravis. Changes in AChR concentration correlate with the clinical severity of myasthenia gravis following therapy and during therapy with prednisone and immunosuppressants. False-positive AChR antibody results may be found in patients with Eaton-Lambert syndrome.

ACID PHOSPHATASE (SERUM)

Normal range: enzymatic, prostatic 0-5.5 U/L; enzymatic, total 2-12 U/L

Elevated in: carcinoma of prostate, other neoplasms (breast, bone), Paget's disease of bone, hemolysis, multiple myeloma, osteogenesis imperfecta, malignant invasion of bone, Gaucher's disease, myeloproliferative disorders, prostatic palpation or surgery, hyperparathyroidism, liver disease, chronic renal failure, idiopathic thrombocytopenic purpura (ITP)

ACID SERUM TEST; SEE HAM TEST
ACTIVATED CLOTTING TIME (ACT)

Normal: This test is used to determine the dose of protamine sulfate to reverse the effect of heparin as an anticoagulant during angioplasty, cardiac surgery, and hemodialysis. The accepted goal during cardiopulmonary bypass surgery is usually 400 to 500 sec.

ACTIVATED PARTIAL THROMBOPLASTIN TIME (aPTT); SEE PARTIAL THROMBOPLASTIN TIME
ADRENOCORTICOTROPIC HORMONE (ACTH)

Normal: 9-52 pg/mL

Elevated in: Addison's disease, ectopic ACTH-producing tumors, congenital adrenal hyperplasia, Nelson's syndrome, pituitary-dependent Cushing's disease

Decreased in: secondary adrenocortical insufficiency, hypopituitarism, adrenal adenoma or adrenal carcinoma

ALANINE AMINOPEPTIDASE

Normal:

Male: 1.11-1.71 μg/mL

Female: 0.96-1.52 μg/mL

Elevated in: liver or pancreatic disease, ethanol ingestion, use of oral contraceptives, malignancy, tobacco use, pregnancy

Decreased in: abortion

ALANINE AMINOTRANSFERASE (ALT, SGPT)

Normal range:

Male: 10-40 U/L

Female: 8-35 U/L

Elevated in: liver disease (e.g., hepatitis, cirrhosis, Reye's syndrome), alcohol abuse, drug use (e.g., acetaminophen, statins, nonsteroidal antiinflammatory drugs [NSAIDs], antibiotics, anabolic steroids, narcotics, heparin, labetalol, amiodarone, chlorpromazine, phenytoin), hepatic congestion, infectious mononucleosis, liver metastases, myocardial infarction [MI], myocarditis, severe muscle trauma, dermatomyositis or polymyositis, muscular dystrophy, malignancy, renal and pulmonary infarction, convulsions, eclampsia, dehydration (relative increase), ingestion of Chinese herbs

Decreased in: azotemia, malnutrition, advanced, chronic renal dialysis, chronic alcoholic liver disease, metronidazole use

ALBUMIN (SERUM)

Normal range: 4-6 g/dl

Elevated in: dehydration (relative increase), IV albumin infusion

Decreased in: liver disease, nephrotic syndrome, poor nutritional status, rapid intravenous (IV) hydration, protein-losing enteropathies (inflammatory bowel disease), severe burns, neoplasia, chronic inflammatory diseases, pregnancy, prolonged immobilization, lymphomas, hypervitaminosis A, chronic glomerulonephritis

ALCOHOL DEHYDROGENASE

Normal: 0-7 U/L

Elevated in: drug-induced hepatocellular damage, obstructive jaundice, malignancy, inflammation, infection

ALDOLASE (SERUM)

Normal range: 0-6 U/L

Elevated in: rhabdomyolysis, dermatomyositis or polymyositis, trichinosis, acute hepatitis and other liver diseases, muscular dystrophy, MI, prostatic carcinoma, hemorrhagic pancreatitis, gangrene, delirium tremens, burns

Decreased in: loss of muscle mass, late stages of muscular dystrophy

ALDOSTERONE (PLASMA)

Normal:

Adult supine: 3-16 ng/dL
Adult upright: 7-30 ng/dL
Adrenal vein: 200-800 ng/dL

Elevated in: aldosterone-secreting adenoma, bilateral adrenal hyperplasia, secondary aldosteronism (diuretics, congestive heart failure [CHF], laxatives, nephritic syndrome, cirrhosis with ascites, Bartter's syndrome, pregnancy, starvation

Decreased in: Addison's disease, rennin deficiency, Turner's syndrome, diabetes mellitus (DM), isolated aldosterone deficiency, post-acute alcohol intoxication (hangover phase)

ALKALINE PHOSPHATASE (SERUM)

Normal range: 30-120 U/L

Elevated in: biliary obstruction, cirrhosis (particularly primary biliary cirrhosis), liver disease (hepatitis, infiltrative liver diseases, fatty metamorphosis), Paget's disease of bone, osteitis deformans, rickets, osteomalacia, hypervitaminosis D, hyperparathyroidism, hyperthyroidism, ulcerative colitis, bowel perforation, bone metastases, healing fractures, bone neoplasms, acromegaly, infectious mononucleosis, cytomegalovirus (CMV) infections, sepsis, pulmonary infarction, hypernephroma, leukemia, myelofibrosis, multiple myeloma, drug therapy (estrogens, albumin, erythromycin and other antibiotics, cholestasis-producing drugs [phenothiazines]), pregnancy, puberty, postmenopausal females

Decreased in: hypothyroidism, pernicious anemia, hypophosphatemia, hypervitaminosis D, malnutrition

ALPHA-1-ANTITRYPSIN (SERUM)

Normal range: 110-140 mg/dL
Decreased in: homozygous or heterozygous deficiency

ALPHA-1-FETOPROTEIN (SERUM)

Normal range: 0-20 ng/ml
Elevated in: hepatocellular carcinoma (usual values >1000 ng/ml), germinal neoplasms (testis, ovary, mediastinum, retroperitoneum), liver disease (alcoholic cirrhosis, acute hepatitis, chronic active hepatitis), fetal anencephaly, spina bifida, basal cell carcinoma, breast carcinoma, pancreatic carcinoma, gastric carcinoma, retinoblastoma, esophageal atresia

ALT; SEE ALANINE AMINOTRANSFERASE
ALUMINUM (SERUM)

Normal range: 0-6 ng/mL
Elevated in: chronic renal failure on dialysis, parenteral nutrition, industrial exposure

AMA; SEE MITOCHONDRIAL ANTIBODY
AMEBIASIS SEROLOGICAL TEST

Test description: Test is used to support diagnosis of amebiasis caused by *Entamoeba histolytica*. Serum acute and convalescent titers are drawn 1 to 3 weeks apart. A fourfold increase in titer is the most indicative result.

AMINOLEVULIC ACID (d-ALA) (24-HOUR URINE COLLECTION)

Normal: 1.5-7.5 md/day
Elevated in: acute porphyrias, lead poisoning, DKA, pregnancy, use of anticonvulsant drugs, hereditary tyrosinemia
Decreased in: alcoholic liver disease

AMMONIA (SERUM)

Normal range:
Adults: 15-45 µg/dl
Children: 29-70 µg/dl
Elevated in: hepatic failure, hepatic encephalopathy, Reye's syndrome, portacaval shunt, drug therapy (diuretics, polymyxin B, methicillin)
Decreased in: drug therapy (neomycin, lactulose), renal failure

AMYLASE (SERUM)

Normal range: 0-130 U/L
Elevated in: acute pancreatitis, macroamylasemia, salivary gland inflammation, mumps, pancreatic neoplasm, abscess, pseudocyst, ascites, perforated peptic ulcer, intestinal obstruction, intestinal infarction, acute cholecystitis, appendicitis, ruptured ectopic pregnancy, peritonitis, burns, diabetic ketoacidosis, renal insufficiency, drug use (morphine), carcinomatosis of lung, esophagus, ovary, acute ethanol ingestion, prostate tumors, post–endoscopic retrograde cholangiopancreatography (ERCP), bulimia, anorexia nervosa
Decreased in: advanced chronic pancreatitis, hepatic necrosis, cystic fibrosis

AMYLASE, URINE; SEE URINE AMYLASE
AMYLOID A PROTEIN (SERUM)

Normal: <10 mcg/mL
Elevated in: inflammatory disorders (acute phase-reacting protein), infections, acute coronary syndrome, malignancies

ANA; SEE ANTINUCLEAR ANTIBODY
ANCA; SEE ANTINEUTROPHIL CYTOPLASMIC ANTIBODY
ANDROSTENEDIONE (SERUM)
Normal:
  Male: 75-205 ng/dL
  Female: 85-275 ng/dL
  Elevated in: congenital adrenal hyperplasia, polycystic ovary syndrome, ectopic ACTH-producing tumor, Cushing's syndrome, hirsutism, hyperplasia of ovarian stroma, ovarian neoplasm
  Decreased in: ovarian failure, adrenal failure, sickle cell anemia

ANGIOTENSIN II
  Normal: 10-60 pg/mL
  Elevated in: hypertension, CHF, cirrhosis, renin-secreting renal tumor, volume depletion
  Decreased in: angiotensin-converting enzyme (ACE) inhibitor drugs, angiotensin II receptor blocker (ARB) drugs, primary aldosteronism, Cushing's syndrome

ANGIOTENSIN-CONVERTING ENZYME (ACE LEVEL)
  Normal range: <40 nmol/ml/min
  Elevated in: sarcoidosis, primary biliary cirrhosis, alcoholic liver disease, hyperthyroidism, hyperparathyroidism, diabetes mellitus, amyloidosis, multiple myeloma, lung disease (asbestosis, silicosis, berylliosis, allergic alveolitis, coccidioidomycosis), Gaucher's disease, leprosy
  Decreased in: ACE inhibitor therapy

ANH; SEE ATRIAL NATRIURETIC HORMONE
ANION GAP
  Normal range: 9-14 mEq/L
  Elevated in: lactic acidosis, ketoacidosis (DKA, alcoholic starvation), uremia (chronic renal failure), ingestion of toxins (paraldehyde, methanol, salicylates, ethylene glycol), hyperosmolar nonketotic coma, antibiotic therapy (carbenicillin)
  Decreased in: hypoalbuminemia, severe hypermagnesemia, IgG myeloma, lithium toxicity, laboratory error (falsely decreased sodium or overestimation of bicarbonate or chloride), hypercalcemia of parathyroid origin, antibiotic therapy (e.g., polymyxin)

ANTICARDIOLIPIN ANTIBODY (ACA)
  Normal range: negative. Test includes detection of IgG, IgM, and IgA antibody to phospholipid, cardiolipin
  Present in: antiphospholipid antibody syndrome, chronic hepatitis C

ANTICOAGULANT; SEE CIRCULATING ANTICOAGULANT
ANTI-HCV; SEE HEPATITIS C ANTIBODY
ANTIDIURETIC HORMONE
  Normal: mOsm/kg 295-300; 4-12 pg/ml
  Elevated in: syndrome of inappropriate antidiuretic hormone (SIADH), antipsychotic medication therapy, ectopic antidiuretic hormone (ADH) from systemic neoplasm, Guillain-Barré, central nervous system (CNS) infections, brain tumors, nephrogenic diabetes insipidus
  Decreased in: central diabetes insipidus, nephritic syndrome, psychogenic polydypsia, demeclocycline, lithium therapy, phenytoin use, alcohol use

ANTI-DNA
Normal range: absent
Present in: systemic lupus erythematosus (SLE), chronic active hepatitis, infectious mononucleosis, biliary cirrhosis

ANTI-ds DNA
Normal: <25 U
Elevated in: systemic lupus erythematosus

ANTI-GLOBIN TEST, DIRECT; SEE COOMBS TEST, DIRECT
ANTIGLOMERULAR BASEMENT ANTIBODY; SEE GLOMERULAR BASEMENT MEMBRANE ANTIBODY

ANTIHISTONE
Normal: <1 U
Elevated in: drug-induced lupus erythematosus

ANTIMITOCHONDRIAL ANTIBODY (AMA)
Normal range: <1:20 titer
Elevated in: primary biliary cirrhosis (85%-95%), chronic active hepatitis (25%-30%), cryptogenic cirrhosis (25%-30%)

ANTINEUTROPHIL CYTOPLASMIC ANTIBODY (ANCA)
Positive test: Cytoplasmic pattern (cANCA): positive in Wegener's granulomatosis
Perinuclear pattern (pANCA): positive in inflammatory bowel disease, primary biliary cirrhosis, primary sclerosing cholangitis, autoimmune chronic active hepatitis, crescenteric glomerulonephritis

ANTINUCLEAR ANTIBODY (ANA)
Normal range: <1:20 titer
Positive test: SLE (more significant if titer > 1:160), drug therapy (phenytoin, ethosuximide, primidone, methyldopa, hydralazine, carbamazepine, penicillin, procainamide, chlorpromazine, griseofulvin, thiazides), chronic active hepatitis, age over 60 years (particularly age over 80), rheumatoid arthritis, scleroderma, mixed connective tissue disease, necrotizing vasculitis, Sjögren's syndrome (SS)
Figure 2-1 describes diagnostic tests and diagnoses to consider from ANA pattern.

ANTIPHOSPHOLIPID ANTIBODY; SEE LUPUS ANTICOAGULANT
ANTI-RNP ANTIBODY; SEE EXTRACTABLE NUCLEAR ANTIGEN
ANTI-Scl-70
Normal: absent
Elevated in: scleroderma

ANTI-Sm (ANTI-SMITH) ANTIBODY; SEE EXTRACTABLE NUCLEAR ANTIGEN
ANTI-SMOOTH MUSCLE ANTIBODY; SEE SMOOTH MUSCLE ANTIBODY
ANTISTREPTOLYSIN O TITER (STREPTOZYME, ASLO TITER)
Normal range for adults: <160 Todd units
Elevated in: streptococcal upper airway infection, acute rheumatic fever, acute glomerulonephritis, increased levels of ß-lipoprotein (false-positive ASLO test)

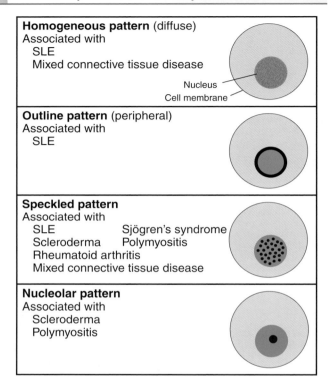

Figure 2-1 Patterns of immunofluorescent staining of antinuclear antibodies and the diseases with which they are associated. *(From Pagana KD, Pagana TJ: Mosby's Diagnostic and Laboratory Test Reference, ed 8, St. Louis, Mosby, 2007.)*

Note: A fourfold increase in titer between acute and convalescent specimens is diagnostic of streptococcal upper airway infection regardless of the initial titer.

ANTITHROMBIN III
Normal range: 81% to 120% of normal activity; 17-30 mg/dl
Decreased in: hereditary deficiency of antithrombin III, disseminated intravascular coagulation (DIC), pulmonary embolism, cirrhosis, thrombolytic therapy, chronic liver failure, postsurgery, third trimester of pregnancy, oral contraceptive use, nephrotic syndrome, IV heparin therapy > 3 days, sepsis, acute leukemia, carcinoma, thrombophlebitis
Elevated in: warfarin drug therapy, post-MI

APOLIPOPROTEIN A-1 (Apo A-1)
Normal: Recommended >120 mg/dl

Elevated in: familial hyperalphalipoproteinemia, statins, niacin, estrogens, weight loss, familial cholesteryl ester transfer protein (CETP) deficiency

Decreased in: familial hypoalphalipoproteinemia, Tangier disease, diuretic use, androgens, cigarette smoking, hepatocellular disorders, chronic renal failure, nephritic syndrome, coronary heart disease, cholestasis

APOLIPOPROTEIN B (Apo B)

Normal: desirable < 100 mg/dL, high risk > 120 mg/dl

Elevated in: high saturated fat diet, high-cholesterol diethyperapobetalipoproteinemia, familial combined hyperlipidemia, anabolic steroids, diuretic use, beta blockers therapy, corticosteroid use, progestin use, diabetes, hypothyroidism, chronic renal failure, liver disease, Cushing's syndrome, coronary heart disease

Decreased in: statin therapy, niacin, low-cholesterol diet, malnutrition, abetalipoproteinemia, hypobetalipoproteinemia, hyperthyroidism

ARTERIAL BLOOD GASES

Normal range:
Po_2: 75-100 mm Hg
Pco_2: 35-45 mm Hg
HCO_3: 24-28 mEq/L
pH: 7.35-7.45
Abnormal values: Acid-base disturbances (see below)

1. Metabolic acidosis
   a. Metabolic acidosis with increased Anion Gap (AG) (AG acidosis)
      1. Lactic acidosis
      2. Ketoacidosis (diabetes mellitus, alcoholic ketoacidosis)
      3. Uremia (chronic renal failure).
      4. Ingestion of toxins (paraldehyde, methanol, salicylate, ethylene glycol)
      5. High-fat diet (mild acidosis)
   b. Metabolic acidosis with normal AG (hyperchloremic acidosis)
      1. Renal tubular acidosis (including acidosis of aldosterone deficiency)
      2. Intestinal loss of HCO_3^- (diarrhea, pancreatic fistula)
      3. Carbonic anhydrase inhibitors (e.g., acetazolamide)
      4. Dilutional acidosis (as a result of rapid infusion of bicarbonate-free isotonic saline)
      5. Ingestion of exogenous acids (ammonium chloride, methionine, cystine, calcium chloride)
      6. Ileostomy
      7. Ureterosigmoidostomy
      8. Drug therapy: amiloride, triamterene, spironolactone, beta blockers
2. Respiratory acidosis
   a. Pulmonary disease (chronic obstructive pulmonary disease [COPD], severe pneumonia, pulmonary edema, interstitial fibrosis)
   b. Airway obstruction (foreign body, severe bronchospasm, laryngospasm)
   c. Thoracic cage disorders (pneumothorax, flail chest, kyphoscoliosis)
   d. Defects in muscles of respiration (myasthenia gravis, hypokalemia, muscular dystrophy)
   e. Defects in peripheral nervous system (amyotrophic lateral sclerosis, poliomyelitis, Guillain-Barré syndrome, botulism, tetanus, organophosphate poisoning, spinal cord injury)
   f. Depression of respiratory center (anesthesia, narcotics, sedatives, vertebral artery embolism or thrombosis, increased intracranial pressure)
   g. Failure of mechanical ventilator
3. Metabolic alkalosis

It is divided into chloride-responsive (urinary chloride < 15 mEq/L) and chloride-resistant forms (urinary chloride level > 15 mEq/L).

  a. Chloride-responsive
     1. Vomiting
     2. Nasogastric (NG) suction
     3. Diuretics
     4. Posthypercapnic alkalosis
     5. Stool losses (laxative abuse, cystic fibrosis, villous adenoma)
     6. Massive blood transfusion
     7. Exogenous alkali administration
  b. Chloride-resistant
     1. Hyperadrenocorticoid states (Cushing's syndrome, primary hyperaldosteronism, secondary mineralocorticoidism [licorice ingestion, chewing tobacco use])
     2. Hypomagnesemia
     3. Hypokalemia
     4. Bartter's syndrome
4. Respiratory alkalosis
     1. Hypoxemia (pneumonia, pulmonary embolism, atelectasis, high-altitude living)
     2. Drugs (salicylates, xanthines, progesterone, epinephrine, thyroxine, nicotine)
     3. CNS disorders (tumor, cerebrovascular accident [CVA], trauma, infections)
     4. Psychogenic hyperventilation (anxiety, hysteria)
     5. Hepatic encephalopathy
     6. Gram-negative sepsis
     7. Hyponatremia
     8. Sudden recovery from metabolic acidosis
     9. Assisted ventilation

ARTHROCENTESIS FLUID

Interpretation of results:

1. **Color**: Normally it is clear or pale yellow; cloudiness indicates inflammatory process or presence of crystals, cell debris, fibrin, or triglycerides.

2. **Viscosity**: Normally it has a high viscosity because of hyaluronate; when fluid is placed on a slide, it can be stretched to a string greater than 2 cm in length before separating (low viscosity indicates breakdown of hyaluronate [lysosomal enzymes from leukocytes] or the presence of edema fluid).

3. **Mucin clot**: Add 1 ml of fluid to 5 ml of a 5% acetic acid solution and allow 1 minute for the clot to form; a firm clot (does not fragment on shaking) is normal and indicates the presence of large molecules of hyaluronic acid (this test is nonspecific and infrequently done).

4. **Glucose**: Normally it approximately equals serum glucose level; a difference of more than 40 mg/dl is suggestive of infection.

5. **Protein**: Total protein concentration is less than 2.5 g/dl in the normal synovial fluid; it is elevated in inflammatory and septic arthritis.

6. **Microscopic examination for crystals**
     a. Gout: monosodium urate crystals
     b. Pseudogout: calcium pyrophosphate dihydrate crystals

Table 2-1 describes synovial fluid findings in common disorders.

ASLO TITER; SEE ANTISTREPTOLYSIN O TITER

ASPARTATE AMINOTRANSFERASE (AST, SGOT)

Normal range: 0-35 U/L

TABLE 2-1 Knee Joint Synovial Fluid Findings in Common Forms of Arthritis

	Normal	Osteoarthritis	Rheumatoid and Other Inflammatory Arthritis	Septic Arthritis
Gross appearance	Clear	Clear	Opaque	Opaque
Volume (ml)	0-1	0-10	5-50	5-50
Viscosity	High	High	Low	Low
Total white cell count/mm^3	<200	200-10,000	500-75,000	>50,000
%polymorphonu-clear cells	<25	<50	>50	>75

From Hochberg MC et al, eds: *Rheumatology*, ed 3, St. Louis, Mosby, 2003.

Elevated in: liver disease (hepatitis, hemochromatosis, cirrhosis, Reye's syndrome, Wilson's disease), alcohol abuse, drug therapy (acetaminophen, statins, NSAIDs, ACE inhibitors, heparin, labetalol, phenytoin, amiodarone, chlorpromazine), hepatic congestion, infectious mononucleosis, MI, myocarditis, severe muscle trauma, dermatomyositis/polymyositis, muscular dystrophy, malignancy, renal and pulmonary infarction, convulsions, eclampsia

Decreased in: uremia, vitamin B_6 deficiency

ATRIAL NATRIURETIC HORMONE (ANH)
Normal: 20-77 pg/ml
Elevated in: CHF, volume overload, cardiovascular disease with high filling pressure
Decreased with: prazosin use

BASOPHIL COUNT
Normal range: 0.4% to 1% of total white blood cells (WBCs); 40-100/mm^3
Elevated in: inflammatory processes, leukemia, polycythemia vera, Hodgkin's lymphoma, hemolytic anemia, after splenectomy, myeloid metaplasia, myxedema
Decreased in: stress, hypersensitivity reaction, steroids, pregnancy, hyperthyroidism

BICARBONATE
Normal:
   Arterial: 21-28 mEq/L
   Venous: 22-29 mEq/L
Elevated in: metabolic alkalosis, compensated respiratory acidosis, diuretics, corticosteroids, laxative abuse
Decreased in: metabolic acidosis; compensated respiratory alkalosis; acetazolamide, cyclosporine, or cholestyramine use; methanol or ethylene glycol poisoning

BILE ACID BREATH TEST
Normal: The test determines the radioactivity of $^{14}CO_2$ in breath samples at 2 and 4 hours.
   2 hours after dose: 0.11 +/− 0.14
   4 hours after dose: 0.52 +/0.09
Elevated in: gastrointestinal (GI) bacterial overgrowth, cimetidine use

BILE, URINE; SEE URINE BILE
BILIRUBIN, DIRECT (CONJUGATED BILIRUBIN)
Normal range: 0-0.2 mg/dl

Elevated in: hepatocellular disease, biliary obstruction, drug-induced cholestasis, hereditary disorders (Dubin-Johnson syndrome, Rotor's syndrome), advanced neoplastic states

BILIRUBIN, INDIRECT (UNCONJUGATED BILIRUBIN)

Normal range: 0-1.0 mg/dl

Elevated in: hemolysis, liver disease (hepatitis, cirrhosis, neoplasm), hepatic congestion caused by congestive heart failure, hereditary disorders (Gilbert's disease, Crigler-Najjar syndrome)

BILIRUBIN, TOTAL

Normal range: 0-1.0 mg/dl

Elevated in: liver disease (hepatitis, cirrhosis, cholangitis, neoplasm, biliary obstruction, infectious mononucleosis), hereditary disorders (Gilbert's disease, Dubin-Johnson syndrome), drug therapy (steroids, diphenylhydantoin, phenothiazines, penicillin, erythromycin, clindamycin, captopril, amphotericin B, sulfonamides, azathioprine, isoniazid [INH], 5-aminosalicylic acid, allopurinol, methyldopa, indomethacin, halothane, oral contraceptives, procainamide, tolbutamide, labetalol), hemolysis, pulmonary embolism or infarct, hepatic congestion resulting from CHF

BILIRUBIN, URINE; SEE URINE BILE

BLADDER TUMOR–ASSOCIATED ANTIGEN

Normal: ≤14 U/mL. The test is used to detect bladder cancer recurrence. Sensitivity is 57% to 83% and specificity 68% to 72%.

Elevated in: bladder cancer, renal stones, nephritis, urinary tract infection (UTI), hematuria, renal cancer, cystitis, recent bladder or urinary tract trauma

BLEEDING TIME (MODIFIED IVY METHOD)

Normal range: 2-9.5 minutes

Elevated in: thrombocytopenia, capillary wall abnormalities, platelet abnormalities (Bernard-Soulier disease, Glanzmann's disease), drug therapy (aspirin, warfarin, anti-inflammatory medications, streptokinase, urokinase, dextran, β-lactam antibiotics, moxalactam), DIC, cirrhosis, uremia, myeloproliferative disorders, von Willebrand's disease

Comments: The bleeding time test as a method to evaluate suspected hemostatic incompetence has been replaced in many laboratories with the platelet function analysis (PFA)-100 assay. The bleeding time test's ability to predict excessive bleeding in clinical situations such as surgery or invasive diagnostic procedures is poor. It may play a limited residual role in the evaluation of suspected hereditary disorders of hemostasis.

BLOOD VOLUME, TOTAL

Normal: 60-80 mL/Kg

Elevated in: polycythemia vera, pulmonary disease, CHF, renal insufficiency, pregnancy, acidosis, thyrotoxicosis

Decreased in: anemia, hemorrhage, vomiting, diarrhea, dehydration, burns, starvation

BORDETELLA PERTUSSIS SEROLOGY

Test description: polymerase chain reaction (PCR) of nasopharyngeal aspirates or secretions is used to identify *Bordetella pertussis,* the organism responsible for whooping cough.

BRCA-1, BRCA-2

This test involves the detection of carriers of mutations in the gene that are characterized by predisposition to breast and ovarian cancers. Women found to carry the mutation should undergo earlier and more intensive surveillance for breast cancer. Pretest counseling should be provided before genetic testing.

BREATH HYDROGEN TEST

Normal: This test is for bacterial overgrowth. Fasting H_2 excretion is 4.6 +/− 5.1, after lactulose, with an early increase of less than 12. Lactulose usually results in a colonic response more than 30 minutes after ingestion.

Elevated in: A high fasting breath H_2 level and an increase of at least 12 ppm within 30 minutes after lactulose challenge are indicative of bacterial overgrowth in the small intestine. The increase must precede the colonic response.

Fast positives in: accelerated gastric emptying, laxative use

Fast negatives in: use of antibiotics and patients who are nonhydrogen producers

B-TYPE NATRIURETIC PEPTIDE

Normal range: up to 100 µg/L. Natriuretic peptides are secreted to regulate fluid volume, blood pressure, and electrolyte balance. They have activity in both the central and peripheral nervous system. In humans the main source of circulatory BNP is the heart ventricles.

Elevated in: heart failure. This test is useful in the emergency department setting to differentiate heart failure patients from those with chronic obstructive pulmonary disease presenting with dyspnea. Levels are also increased in asymptomatic left ventricular dysfunction, arterial and pulmonary hypertension, cardiac hypertrophy, valvular heart disease, arrhythmia, and acute coronary syndrome.

BUN; SEE UREA NITROGEN
C3; SEE COMPLEMENT C3
C4; SEE COMPLEMENT C4
CA 15-3; SEE CANCER ANTIGEN 15-3
CA 27-29; SEE CANCER ANTIGEN 27-29
CA 72-4; SEE CANCER ANTIGEN 72-4
CA 125; SEE CANCER ANTIGEN 125
CALCITONIN (SERUM)

Normal range: < 100 pg/ml

Elevated in: medullary carcinoma of the thyroid (particularly if level >1500 pg/ml), carcinoma of the breast, apudomas, carcinoids, renal failure, thyroiditis

CALCIUM (SERUM)

Normal range: 8.8-10.3 mg/dl

Abnormal values

Elevated in:

1. Malignancy: increased bone resorption via osteoclast-activating factors, secretion of pituitary hormone (PTH)–like substances, prostaglandin E_2, direct erosion by tumor cells, transforming growth factors, colony-stimulating activity. Hypercalcemia is common in the following neoplasms:
   a. Solid tumors: breast, lung, pancreas, kidneys, ovary
   b. Hematologic cancers: myeloma, lymphosarcoma, adult T-cell lymphoma, Burkitt's lymphoma

2. Hyperparathyroidism: increased bone resorption, GI absorption, and renal absorption. Hyperparathyroidism can be caused by the following conditions:
  a. Parathyroid hyperplasia, adenoma
  b. Hyperparathyroidism or renal failure with secondary hyperparathyroidism
3. Granulomatous disorders: increased GI absorption (e.g., sarcoidosis)
4. Paget's disease: increased bone resorption, seen only during periods of immobilization
5. Vitamin D intoxication, milk-alkali syndrome; increased GI absorption
6. Thiazides: increased renal absorption
7. Other causes: familial hypocalciuric hypercalcemia, thyrotoxicosis, adrenal insufficiency, prolonged immobilization, vitamin A intoxication, recovery from acute renal failure, lithium administration, pheochromocytoma, disseminated SLE

Decreased in:
1. Renal insufficiency: hypocalcemia caused by the following:
  a. Increased calcium deposits in bone and soft tissue secondary to increased serum PO_4 3 level
  b. Decreased production of 1,25-dihydroxyvitamin D
  c. Excessive loss of 25-OHD (nephrotic syndrome)
2. Hypoalbuminemia: Each decrease in serum albumin (g/L) will decrease serum calcium by 0.8 mg/dl but will not change free (ionized) calcium.
3. Vitamin D deficiency
  a. Malabsorption (most common cause)
  b. Inadequate intake
  c. Decreased production of 1,25-dihydroxyvitamin D (vitamin D dependent rickets, renal failure)
  d. Decreased production of 25-OHD (parenchymal liver disease)
  e. Accelerated 25-OHD catabolism (phenytoin, phenobarbital)
  f. End-organ resistance to 1,25-dihydroxyvitamin D
4. Hypomagnesemia: hypocalcemia caused by the following:
  a. Decreased PTH secretion
  b. Inhibition of PTH effect on bone
5. Pancreatitis, hyperphosphatemia, osteoblastic metastases: Hypocalcemia is secondary to increased calcium deposits (bone, abdomen).
6. Pseudohypoparathyroidism (PHP): autosomal recessive disorder characterized by short stature, shortening of metacarpal bones, obesity, and mental retardation. Hypocalcemia is secondary to congenital end-organ resistance to PTH.
7. Idiopathic hypoparathyroidism, surgical removal of parathyroids (e.g., neck surgery)
8. "Hungry bones syndrome": rapid transfer of calcium from plasma into bones after removal of a parathyroid tumor
9. Sepsis
10. Massive blood transfusion (as a result of EDTA in blood)

CALCIUM, URINE; SEE URINE CALCIUM
CANCER ANTIGEN 15-3 (CA 15-3)
Normal: <30 U/ml
Elevated in: approximately 80% of women with metastatic breast cancer. Clinical sensitivity is 0.60, specificity 0.87, positive predictive value 0.91. This test is generally used to predict recurrence of breast cancer and evaluate response to therapy. May also be elevated in liver cancer, pancreatic cancer, ovarian cancer, colorectal cancer. Elevations can also occur with benign breast and liver disease

CANCER ANTIGEN 27-29 (CA 27-29)
Normal: <38 U/ml

Elevated in: approximately 75% of women with metastatic breast cancer. Clinical sensitivity is 0.57, specificity 0.97, positive predictive value 0.83, negative predictive value 0.92. This test is generally used to predict recurrence of breast cancer and evaluate response to therapy. May also be elevated in liver cancer, pancreatic cancer, ovarian cancer, colorectal cancer. Elevations can also occur with benign breast and liver disease.

CANCER ANTIGEN 72-4 (CA 72-4)
Normal: <4.0 ng/ml
Elevated in: gastric cancer (elevated in > 50% of patients). Often used in combination with CA 72-4, CA 19-9, and CEA to monitor gastric cancer after treatment.

CANCER ANTIGEN 125 (CA-125)
Normal range: <35 U/ml
Elevated in: epithelial ovarian cancer; carcinoma of fallopian tube and endometrium; nonovarian abdominal malignancies; all forms of liver disease, especially those with cirrhotic ascites

CAPTOPRIL STIMULATION TEST
Normal: This test is performed by giving 25 mg captopril orally after overnight fast. The patient should be seated during the test. After captopril administration, aldosterone is less than 15 ng/dl, renin greater than 2 ng Al/mL/hr.
Interpretation: In patients with primary aldosteronism, plasma aldosterone remains high and plasma renin activity remains low after captopril adminsitration.

CARBAMAZEPINE (TEGRETOL)
Normal therapeutic range: 4-12 µg/ml

CARBOHYDRATE ANTIGEN 19-9
Normal: <37.0 U/ml
Elevated in: GI cancer, most commonly pancreatic cancer. The amount of elevation has no relation to tumor mass. Elevations can also occur with cirrhosis, cholangitis, and chronic or acute pancreatitis.

CARBON DIOXIDE, PARTIAL PRESSURE
Normal:
  Male: 35-48 mm Hg
  Female: 32-45 mm Hg
  Elevated in: respiratory acidosis
  Decreased in: respiratory alkalosis

CARBON MONOXIDE; SEE CARBOXYHEMOGLOBIN
CARBOXYHEMOGLOBIN
Normal range: saturation of hemoglobin <2%; smokers <9% (coma: 50%; death: 80%)
Elevated in: smoking, exposure to smoking, exposure to automobile exhaust fumes, malfunctioning gas-burning appliances

CARDIAC MARKERS (SERUM)
Figure 2-2 describes typical cardiac marker diagnostic window curves and serum levels after myocardial infarction.

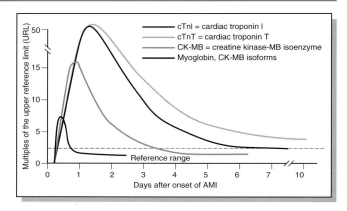

Figure 2-2 Typical cardiac marker diagnostic window curves and serum levels after acute MI. *(From Lehmann CA, ed: Saunders Manual of Clinical Laboratory Science, Philadelphia, WB Saunders, 1998.)*

CARDIAC TROPONINS; SEE TROPONINS
CARCINOEMBRYONIC ANTIGEN (CEA)

Normal range: nonsmokers: 0-2.5 ng/ml; smokers: 0-5 ng/ml
Elevated in: colorectal carcinomas, pancreatic carcinomas, and metastatic disease usually produce higher elevations (>20 ng/ml); carcinomas of the esophagus, stomach, small intestine, liver, breast, ovary, lung, and thyroid usually produce lesser elevations; benign conditions (smoking, inflammatory bowel disease, hypothyroidism, cirrhosis, pancreatitis, infections) usually produce levels less than 10 ng/ml.

CARDIO-CRP; SEE C-REACTIVE PROTEIN
CAROTENE (SERUM)

Normal range: 50-250 µg/dl
Elevated in: carotenemia, chronic nephritis, diabetes mellitus, hypothyroidism, nephrotic syndrome, hyperlipidemia
Decreased in: fat malabsorption, steatorrhea, pancreatic insufficiency, lack of carotenoids in diet, high fever, liver disease

CATECHOLAMINES, URINE; SEE URINE CATECHOLAMINES
CBC; SEE COMPLETE BLOOD CELL COUNT
CCK; SEE CHOLECYSTOKININ-PANCREOZYMIN
CCK-PZ; SEE CHOLECYSTOKININ-PANCREOZYMIN
CD4 T-LYMPHOCYTE COUNT (CD4 T-CELLS)

Calculated as total WBC × % lymphocytes × % lymphocytes stained with CD4.
This test is used primarily to evaluate immune dysfunction in HIV infection and should be done every 3-6 months in all HIV-infected persons. It is useful as a prognostic indicator and as a criterion for initiating prophylaxis for several opportunistic infections that are sequelae of HIV infection. Progressive depletion of CD4 T-lymphocytes is associated with an increased likelihood of clinical

complications. Adolescents and adults with HIV are classified as having acquired immunodeficiency syndrome (AIDS) if their CD4 lymphocyte count is under $200/\mu l$ and/or if their CD4 T-lymphocyte percentage is less than 14%. HIV-infected patients whose CD4 count is less than $200/\mu l$ and who acquire certain infectious diseases or malignancies are also classified as having AIDS. Corticosteroids decrease CD4 T-cell percentage and absolute number.

CD40 LIGAND

Normal: $<5 \mu g/L$. CD40 ligand is a soluble protein that is shed from activated leukocytes and platelets and used in risk stratification for acute coronary syndrome.

Elevated in: acute coronary syndrome. Increased CD40 ligand is associated with higher incidence of death or nonfatal MI.

CEA; SEE CARCINOEMBRYONIC ANTIGEN
CEREBROSPINAL FLUID (CSF)

Normal range:
  Appearance: clear
  Glucose: 40-70 mg/dl
  Protein: 20-45 mg/dl
  Chloride: 116-122 mEq/L
  Pressure: 100-200 mm H_2O
  Cell count (cells/mm³) and cell type: <6 lymphocytes, no polymorphonucleocytes

Interpretation of results:
1. Appearance of the fluid:
   a. Clear fluid indicates that results are normal.
   b. Yellow (xanthochromia) in the supernatant of centrifuged CSF within 1 hour or less after collection is usually the result of previous bleeding (subarachnoid hemorrhage); it may also be caused by increased CSF protein, melanin from meningeal melanosarcomas, or carotenoids.
   c. Pinkish color is usually the result of a bloody tap; the color generally clears progressively from tubes 1 to 4 (the supernatant is usually crystal clear in traumatic taps).
   d. Turbidity usually indicates the presence of leukocytes (bleeding introduces approximately 1 WBC/500 red blood cells [RBCs] into the CSF).
2. CSF pressure: Elevated pressure can be seen with meningitis, meningoencephalitis, pseudotumor cerebri, mass lesions, and intracerebral bleeding.
3. Cell count: In adults the CSF is normally free of cells (although up to 5 mononuclear cells/mm³ is considered normal); the presence of granulocytes is never normal.
   a. Neutrophils: These are seen in bacterial meningitis, early viral meningoencephalitis, and early tuberculosis (TB) meningitis.
   b. Increased lymphocytes are seen in TB meningitis, viral meningoencephalitis, syphilitic meningoencephalitis, fungal meningitis.
4. Protein: Serum proteins are generally too large to cross the normal blood-CSF barrier; however, increased CSF protein is seen with meningeal inflammation, traumatic tap, increased CNS synthesis, tissue degeneration, obstruction to CSF circulation, and Guillain-Barré syndrome.
5. Glucose:
   a. Decreased glucose is seen with bacterial meningitis, TB meningitis, fungal meningitis, subarachnoid hemorrhage, and some cases of viral meningitis.
   b. A mild increase in CSF glucose can be seen in patients with very elevated serum glucose levels.

CERULOPLASMIN (SERUM)

Normal range: 20-35 mg/dl

Elevated in: pregnancy, estrogen therapy, oral contraceptive use, neoplastic diseases (leukemias, Hodgkin's lymphoma, carcinomas), inflammatory states, SLE, primary biliary cirrhosis, rheumatoid arthritis

Decreased in: Wilson's disease (values often <10 mg/dl), nephrotic syndrome, advanced liver disease, malabsorption, total parenteral nutrition, Menkes' syndrome

CHLAMYDIA GROUP ANTIBODY SEROLOGIC TEST

Test description: Acute and convalescent sera is drawn 2 to 4 weeks apart. A fourfold increase in titer between acute and convalescent sera is necessary for confirmation. A single titer 1:64 or higher is considered indicative of psittacosis or lymphogranuloma venereum (LGV).

CHLAMYDIA TRACHOMATIS PCR

Test description: Performed on endocervical swab, urine, and intraurethral swab

CHLORIDE (SERUM)

Normal range: 95-105 mEq/L

Elevated in: dehydration, sodium loss greater than chloride loss, respiratory alkalosis, excessive infusion of normal saline solution, cystic fibrosis, hyperparathyroidism, renal tubular disease, metabolic acidosis, prolonged diarrhea, acetazolamide administration, diabetes insipidus, ureterosigmoidostomy

Decreased in: vomiting, gastric suction, primary aldosteronism, CHF, SIADH, Addison's disease, salt-losing nephritis, continuous infusion of D_5W, thiazide diuretic administration, diaphoresis, diarrhea, burns, DKA

CHLORIDE (SWEAT)

Normal: 0-40 mmol/L

Borderline/indeterminate: 41-60 mmol/L

Consistent with cystic fibrosis: >60 mmol/L

False low results can occur with edema, excessive sweating, and hypoproteinemia.

CHLORIDE, URINE; SEE URINE CHLORIDE
CHOLECYSTOKININ-PANCREOZYMIN (CCK, CCK-PZ)

Normal: < 80 pg/ml

Elevated in: pancreatic disease, celiac disease, gastric ulcer, postgastrectomy state, irritable bowel syndrome (IBS), fatty food intolerance

CHOLESTEROL, LOW-DENSITY LIPOPROTEIN; SEE LOW-DENSITY LIPOPROTEIN CHOLESTEROL
CHOLESTEROL, HIGH-DENSITY LIPOPROTEIN; SEE HIGH-DENSITY LIPOPROTEIN CHOLESTEROL
CHOLESTEROL, TOTAL

Normal range: Generally <200 mg/dl

Elevated in: primary hypercholesterolemia, biliary obstruction, diabetes mellitus, nephrotic syndrome, hypothyroidism, primary biliary cirrhosis, diet high in cholesterol and total and saturated fat, third trimester of pregnancy, drug therapy (steroids, phenothiazines, oral contraceptives)

Decreased in: use of lipid-lowering agents (statins, niacin, ezetimibe, cholestyramine, colesevelam), starvation, malabsorption, abetalipoproteinemia, hyperthyroidism, hepatic failure, carcinoma, infection, inflammation

CHORIONIC GONADOTROPINS (hCG), HUMAN (SERUM)

Normal range, serum:
  Male: <0.7 IU/L
  Female premenopausal: <0.8 IU/L
  Female postmenopausal: <3.3 IU/L
  Elevated in: pregnancy, choriocarcinoma, gestational trophoblastic neoplasia (including molar gestations), placental site trophoblastic tumors; human antimouse antibodies (HAMA) can produce false serum assay for hCG.

  The principal use of this test is to diagnose pregnancy. In pregnancy the concentration of hCG increases significantly during the initial 6 weeks of pregnancy. Peak values approaching 100,000 IU/L occur 60 to 70 days following implantation.

  hCG levels generally double every 1 to 3 days. In patients with concentration less than 2000 IU/L, an increase of serum hCG less than 66% after 2 days is suggestive of spontaneous abortion or ruptured ectopic gestation.

CHYMOTRYPSIN

Normal: <10 µg/L
  Elevated in: acute pancreatitis, chronic renal failure, oral enzyme preparations, gastric cancer, pancreatic cancer
  Decreased in: chronic pancreatitis, late cystic fibrosis

CIRCULATING ANTICOAGULANT (ANTIPHOSPHOLIPID ANTIBODY, LUPUS ANTICOAGULANT)

Normal: negative
  Detected in: SLE, drug-induced lupus, long-term phenothiazine therapy, multiple myeloma, ulcerative colitis, rheumatoid arthritis, postpartum, hemophilia, neoplasms, chronic inflammatory states, AIDS, nephrotic syndrome
  Note: The name is a misnomer because these patients are prone to hypercoagulability and thrombosis.

CK; SEE CREATINE KINASE

CLONIDINE SUPPRESSION TEST

Interpretation: Clonidine inhibits neurogenic catecholamine release and will cause a decrease in plasma norepinephrine into the reference interval in hypertensive subjects without pheochromocytoma. The test is performed by giving 4.3 µg clonidine/kg orally after overnight fast. Norepinephrine is measured at 3 hours. Result should be within established reference range and decrease to less than 50% of baseline concentration. Lack of decrease in norepinephrine is suggestive of pheochromocytoma.

CLOSTRIDIUM DIFFICILE TOXIN ASSAY (STOOL)

Normal: negative
  Detected in: antibiotic-associated diarrhea and pseudomembranous colitis

CO; SEE CARBOXYHEMOGLOBIN

COAGULATION FACTORS

Factor reference ranges:
  V: >10%
  VII: >10%
  VIII: 50% to 170%
  IX: 60% to 136%
  X: >10%

XI: 50% to 150%
XII: >30%
   Figure 2-3 illustrates the blood coagulation pathways.

COLD AGGLUTININS TITER
   Normal range: <1:32
   Elevated in: primary atypical pneumonia (*Mycoplasma* pneumonia), infectious mononucleosis, CMV infection, others (hepatic cirrhosis, acquired hemolytic anemia, frostbite, multiple myeloma, lymphoma, malaria)

COMPLEMENT (C3, C4)
   Normal range: C3: 70-160 mg/dl; C4: 20-40 mg/dl

   Abnormal values:
   Decreased C3: active SLE, immune complex disease, acute glomerulonephritis, inborn C3 deficiency, membranoproliferative glomerulonephritis, infective endocarditis, serum sickness, autoimmune/chronic active hepatitis
   Decreased C4: immune complex disease, active SLE, infective endocarditis, inborn C4 deficiency, hereditary angioedema, hypergammaglobulinemic states, cryobulinemic vasculitis

COMPLETE BLOOD CELL COUNT (CBC)
   WBCs: 3200-9800/mm^3
   RBCs: 4.3-5.9 10^6/mm^3 (male); 3.5-5.0 10^6/mm^3 (female)
   Hemoglobin: 13.6-17.7 g/dl (male); 12-15 g/dl (female)
   Hematocrit: 39% to 49% (male); 33% to 43% (female)
   MCV: 76-100 μm^3
   MCH: 27-33 pg
   MCHC: 33-37 g/dl
   RDW: 11.5% to 14.5%
   Platelet count: 130-400 × 10^3/mm^3
   Differential: 2-6 bands (early mature neutrophils); 60-70 segs (mature neutrophils); 1-4 eosinophils; 0-1 basophils; 2-8 monocytes; 25-40 lymphocytes

CONJUGATED BILIRUBIN; SEE BILIRUBIN, DIRECT
COOMBS, DIRECT (ANTIGLOBULIN TEST, DIRECT, DAT)
   Normal: negative
   Positive: (Figure 2-4) autoimmune hemolytic anemia, erythroblastosis fetalis, transfusion reactions, drug therapy (methyldopa, penicillins, tetracycline, sulfonamides, levodopa, cephalosporins, quinidine, insulin)
   False positive: may be seen with cold agglutinins

COOMBS, INDIRECT
   Normal: negative
   Positive: (Figure 2-5) acquired hemolytic anemia, incompatible cross-matched blood, anti-Rh antibodies, drug therapy (methyldopa, mefenamic acid, levodopa)

CPK; SEE CREATINE KINASE
COPPER (SERUM)
   Normal range: 70-140 μg/dl
   Decreased in: Wilson's disease, malabsorption, malnutrition, nephrosis, total parenteral nutrition (TPN), acute leukemia in remission

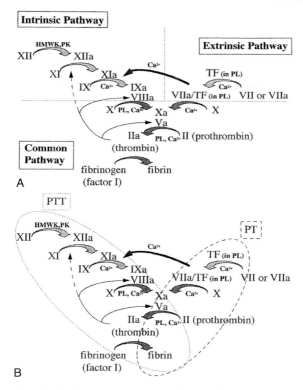

Figure 2-3 Simplified coagulation cascade. **A,** The coagulation cascade has historically been divided into two main pathways—the intrinsic and extrinsic pathways—both of which culminate in the formation of fibrin through the common pathway. It is now believed that factor IX activation by the factor VIIa/TF complex plays a major role in the initiation of normal hemostasis. Once coagulation is activated, factor Xa binds to the tissue factor pathway inhibitor (TFPI), which then effectively inhibits factor VIIa/TF. The factor VIIIa/IXa complex becomes the dominant generator of factor Xa and thus thrombin and fibrin formation. This model is consistent with the observation that deficiencies in factors VIII, IX, and to a lesser extent XI cause a bleeding diathesis, whereas the absence of factor XII, PK, or HMWK does not. In the intrinsic pathway, factor XIIa activates prekallikrein into kallikrein. Kallikrein then activates more factor XIIa from factor XII. HMWK acts as a cofactor in both these reactions. HMWK also acts as a cofactor in the activation of factor XI by factor XII. Kallikrein releases bradykinin from HMWK, which has vasoactive activities. **B,** The aPTT measures the clotting time from factor XII through fibrin formation. The prothrombin time (PT) measures the clotting time from factor VII through fibrin formation. (Ca^2, calcium; *HMWK,* high-molecular-weight kininogen; *PK,* prekallikrein; *PL,* phospholipid;. *TF,* tissue factor [a transmembrane protein; thus, it is associated with phospholipid in vivo].) *(From Henry JB, ed: Clinical Diagnosis and Management by Laboratory Methods, Philadelphia, WB Saunders, 2001.)*

DIRECT COOMBS TEST

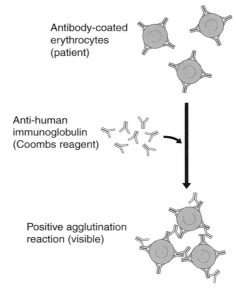

Antibody-coated
erythrocytes
(patient)

Anti-human
immunoglobulin
(Coombs reagent)

Positive agglutination
reaction (visible)

Figure 2-4 Positive direct Coombs test (direct antiglobulin test). Anti-human immunoglobulin (reagent) is added to the patient's red blood cells, which have been coated with antibody (in vivo). The reagent anti-human immunoglobulin attaches to the antibodies coating the patient's red blood cells, causing visible agglutination. *(From Young NS, Gerson SL, High KA, eds: Clinical Hematology, St. Louis, Mosby, 2006.)*

Elevated in: aplastic anemia, biliary cirrhosis, SLE, hemochromatosis, hyperthyroidism, hypothyroidism, infection, iron deficiency anemia, leukemia, lymphoma, oral contraceptive use, pernicious anemia, rheumatoid arthritis

COPPER, URINE; SEE URINE COPPER
CORTICOTROPIN-RELEASING HORMONE (CRH) STIMULATION TEST

Normal: A dose of 0.5 mg of dexamethasone is given every 6 hours for 2 days; 2 hours after last dose 1 µg/kg CRH is given intravenously. Samples are drawn after 15 minutes. Normally there is a twofold to fourfold increase in mean baseline concentration of ACTH or cortisol. Cortisol greater than 1.4 µg/L is virtually 100% specific and 100% diagnostic.

Interpretation: Normal or exaggerated response: pituitary Cushing's disease
No response: ectopic ACTH-secreting tumor
A positive response to CRH or a suppressed response to high-dose dexamethasone has a 97% positive predictive value for Cushing's disease. However, a lack

INDIRECT COOMBS TEST

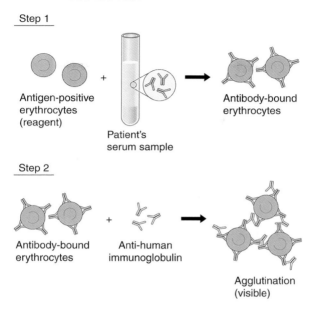

Step 1

Antigen-positive
erythrocytes
(reagent)

Patient's
serum sample

Antibody-bound
erythrocytes

Step 2

Antibody-bound
erythrocytes

Anti-human
immunoglobulin

Agglutination
(visible)

Figure 2-5 Positive indirect Coombs test (indirect antiglobulin test). In step one, reagent red blood cells coated with antigen are added to the patient's serum, which contains antibody. In the presence of antigen-antibody specificity, the antibody from the patient's serum coats the reagent red blood cells (in vitro); this does not result in visible agglutination. In step two, reagent anti-human immunoglobulin is added to the antibody-bound reagent red blood cells. The reagent anti-human immunoglobulin attaches to the antibodies that are coating the reagent red blood cells, causing visible agglutination. *(From Young NS, Gerson SL, High KA, eds: Clinical Hematology, St. Louis, Mosby, 2006.)*

of response to either test excludes Cushing's disease in only 64% to 78% of patients. When the tests are considered together, negative responses from both have a 100% predictive value for ectopic ACTH secretion.

CORTISOL (PLASMA)

Normal range: varies with time of collection (circadian variation):
8 AM: 4-19 μg/dl
4 PM: 2-15 μg/dl
Elevated in: ectopic ACTH production (i.e., oat cell carcinoma of lung), loss of normal diurnal variation, pregnancy, chronic renal failure, iatrogenic, stress, adrenal or pituitary hyperplasia or adenomas
Decreased in: primary adrenocortical insufficiency, anterior pituitary hypofunction, secondary adrenocortical insufficiency, adrenogenital syndromes

C-PEPTIDE

Normal range (serum): 0.51-2.70 ng/ml

Elevated in: insulinoma, sulfonylurea administration, type 2 DM, renal failure

Decreased in: type 1 DM, factitious insulin administration

CPK; SEE CREATINE KINASE

C-REACTIVE PROTEIN

Normal range: <1 mg/dl. CRP levels are valuable in the clinical assessment of chronic inflammatory disorders such as rheumatoid arthritis, SLE, vasculitis syndromes, and inflammatory bowel disease.

Elevated in: inflammatory and neoplastic diseases, MI, third trimester of pregnancy (acute-phase reactant), oral contraceptive use. Moderately high CRP concentrations (3-10 mg/L) predict increased risk of myocardial infarction and stroke. Markedly high levels (>10 mg/L) have been shown to predict cardiovascular risk.

Note: High sensitivity C-reactive protein (hs-CRP, cardio-CRP): is used as a cardiac risk marker. It is increased in patients with silent atherosclerosis for a prolonged period before a cardiovascular event and is independent of cholesterol level and other lipoproteins. It can be used to help stratify cardiac risk.

Interpretation of results:

Cardio-CRP Level (mg/L)	Risk
<0.6	Lowest risk
0.7-1.1	Low risk
1.2-1.9	Moderate risk
2.0-3.8	High risk
3.9-4.9	Highest risk
≥5.0	Results may be confounded by acute inflammatory disease. If clinically indicated, a repeat test should be performed in 2 or more weeks.

CREATINE KINASE (CK, CPK)

Normal range: 0-130 U/L

Elevated in: vigorous exercise, intramuscular (IM) injections, MI, myocarditis, rhabdomyolysis, myositis, crush injury/trauma, polymyositis, dermatomyositis, muscular dystrophy, myxedema, seizures, malignant hyperthermia syndrome, CVA, pulmonary embolism and infarction, acute dissection of aorta

Decreased in: steroids, decreased muscle mass, connective tissue disorders, alcoholic liver disease, metastatic neoplasms

CREATINE KINASE ISOENZYMES

CK-MB

Elevated in: MI, myocarditis, pericarditis, muscular dystrophy, cardiac defibrillation, cardiac surgery, extensive rhabdomyolysis, strenuous exercise (e.g., marathon runners), mixed connective tissue disease, cardiomyopathy, hypothermia.

Note: CK-MB exists in the blood in two subforms; MB_2 is released from cardiac cells and converted in the blood in MB_1. Rapid assay of CK-MB subforms can detect MI (CK-MB_2 ≥1.0 U/L, with a ratio of CK-MB_2/CK-MB_1 ≥1.5) within the first 6 hours of onset of symptoms.

CK-MM

Elevated in: crush injury, seizures, malignant hyperthermia syndrome, rhabdomyolysis, myositis, polymyositis, dermatomyositis, vigorous exercise, muscular dystrophy, IM injections, acute dissection of aorta

CK-BB

Elevated in: CVA, subarachnoid hemorrhage, neoplasms (prostate, GI tract, brain, ovary, breast, lung), severe shock, bowel infarction, hypothermia, meningitis

CREATININE (SERUM)

Normal range: 0.6-1.2 mg/dl

Elevated in: renal insufficiency (acute and chronic), decreased renal perfusion (hypotension, dehydration, CHF), rhabdomyolysis, administration of contrast dyes, ketonemia, drug therapy (antibiotics [aminoglycosides, cephalosporins], ACE inhibitors [in patients with renal artery stenosis], diuretics)

Falsely elevated in: DKA, administration of some cephalosporins (e.g., cefoxitin, cephalothin)

Decreased in: decreased muscle mass (including amputees and elderly), pregnancy, prolonged debilitation

CREATININE CLEARANCE

Normal range: 75-124 ml/min

Elevated in: pregnancy, exercise

Decreased in: renal insufficiency, drug therapy (e.g., cimetidine, procainamide, antibiotics, quinidine)

CREATININE, URINE; SEE URINE CREATININE

CRYOGLOBULINS (SERUM)

Normal range: not detectable

Present in: collagen-vascular diseases, chronic active hepatitis, chronic lymphocytic leukemia (CLL), hemolytic anemias, multiple myeloma, Waldenström's macroglobulinemia, Hodgkin's disease

CRYPTOSPORIDIUM ANTIGEN BY EIA (STOOL)

Normal range: not detected

Present in: cryptosporidiosis

CSF; SEE CEREBROSPINAL FLUID

CYSTATIN C

Normal: Cystatin C is a cysteine protease inhibitor that is produced at a constant rate by all nucleated cells. It is freely filtered by the glomerulus and reabsorbed (but not secreted) by the renal tubules with no extrarenal excretion. Its concentration is not affected by diet, muscle mass, or acute inflammation. Normal range when measured by particle-enhanced nephelometric immunoassay (PENIA) is <0.28 mg/L.

Elevated in: renal disorders. Good predictor of the severity of acute tubular necrosis. Cystatin C increases more rapidly than creatinine in the early stages of glomerular filtration rate (GFR) impairment. The cystatin C concentration is an independent risk factor for heart failure in older adults and appears to provide a better measure of risk assessment than the serum creatinine concentration.

CYSTIC FIBROSIS PCR

Test description: Can be performed on whole blood or tissue. Common mutations in the cystic fibrosis transmembrane regulator (CFTR) gene can be used to detect 75% to 80% of mutant alleles.

CYTOMEGALOVIRUS BY PCR

Test description: Can be performed on whole blood, plasma, or tissue. Qualitative PCR is highly sensitive but may not be able to differentiate between latent and active infection.

D-Dimer

Normal range: <0.5 μg/mL

Elevated in: DVT, pulmonary embolism, high levels of rheumatoid factor, activation of coagulation and fibrolytic system from any cause

D-dimer assay by enzyme-linked immunosorbent assay (ELISA) assists in the diagnosis of DVT and pulmonary embolism. This test has significant limitations because it can be elevated whenever the coagulation and fibrinolytic systems are activated and can also be falsely elevated with high rheumatoid factor levels.

DEHYDROEPIANDROSTERONE SULFATE

Normal:
> Males: age 19-30: 125-619 μg/dl
> > age 31-50: 59-452 μg/dl
> > age 51-60: 20-413 μg/dl
> > age 61-83: 10-285 μg/dl
> Females: age 19-30: 29-781 μg/dl
> > age 31-50: 12-379 μg/dl
> > Postmenopausal: 30-260 μg/dl

Elevated in: hirsutism, congenital adrenal hyperplasia, adrenal carcinomas, adrenal adenomas, polycystic ovarian syndrome, ectopic ACTH-producing tumors, Cushing's disease, spironolactone

DEOXYCORTICOSTERONE (11-DEOXYCORTICOSTERONE, DOC), SERUM

Normal: 2-19 ng/dl. Normal secretion is dependent on ACTH and is suppressible by dexamethasone.

Elevated in: androgenital syndromes caused by 17- and 11-hydroxylase deficiencies, pregnancy

Decreased in: preeclampsia

DEXAMETHASONE SUPPRESSION TEST, OVERNIGHT

Normal: This test is performed by giving 1 mg dexamethasone orally at 11 PM and measuring serum cortisol at 8 AM on following morning, normal response is cortisol suppression to less than 3 μg/dl. If a dose of 4 mg dexamethasone is given, cortisol suppression will be to less than 50% of baseline.

Interpretation: Cushing's syndrome (>10 μg/dl), endogenous depression (half of patients suppress test values >5 μg/dl). Most patients with pituitary Cushing's disease demonstrate suppression, whereas patients with adrenal adenoma, carcinoma, and ectopic ACTH-producing tumors do not.

DIHYDROTESTOSTERONE, SERUM, URINE

Normal:
> Serum: Males: 30-85 ng/dl

Females: 4-22 ng/dl
Urine: 24 h:
  Males: 20-50 μg/day
  Females: <8 μg/day
Elevated in: hirsutism
Decreased in: 5-alpha-reductase deficiency, hypogonadism

DISACCHARIDE ABSORPTION TESTS
Normal: This test is used to diagnose malabsorption due to disaccharide deficiency. It is performed by giving disaccharide orally 1 g/kg body weight to a total of 25 g. Blood is drawn at 0, 30, 60, 90, and 120 minutes. Normal response is a change in glucose from fasting value more than 30 mg/dl; results are inconclusive when the increase is 20-30 mg/dl and abnormal when the increase is less than 20 mg/dl. The test can also be performed by measuring air at 0, 30, 60, 90, and 120 minutes. Normal is H_2 more than 20 ppm above baseline level before a colonic response.
Decreased in: disaccharide deficiency (lactose, fructose, sorbitol), celiac disease, sprue, acute gastroenteritis

DOC; SEE DEOXYCORTICOSTERONE
DONATH-LANDSTEINER (D-L) TEST FOR PAROXYSMAL COLD HEMOGLOBINURIA
Normal: no hemolysis
Interpretation: hemolysis indicates presence of bithermic cold hemolysins or Donath-Landsteiner antibodies (D-L Ab).

d-XYLOSE ABSORPTION TEST
Normal range:
Urine: ≥4 g/5 hr (5-hour urine collection in adults ≥12 years [25-g dose])
Serum: ≥25 mg/dl (adult, I h, 25-g dose, normal renal function)
Normal results: In patients with malabsorption, normal results suggest pancreatic disease as a cause of the malabsorption.
Abnormal results: celiac disease, Crohn's disease, tropical sprue, surgical bowel resection, AIDS. False positives can occur with decreased renal function, dehydration/hypovolemia, surgical blind loops, decreased gastric emptying, and vomiting.

DIGOXIN (LANOXIN)
Normal therapeutic range: 0.5-2 ng/ml
Elevated in: impaired renal function; excessive dosing; concomitant use of quinidine, amiodarone, verapamil, fluoxetine, nifedipine

DILANTIN; SEE PHENYTOIN
DOPAMINE
Normal range: 0-175 pg/ml
Elevated in: pheochromocytomas, neuroblastomas, stress, vigorous exercise, ingestion of certain foods (bananas, chocolate, coffee, tea, vanilla)

ELECTROLYTES, URINE; SEE URINE ELECTROLYTES
ELECTROPHORESIS, HEMOGLOBIN; SEE HEMOGLOBIN ELECTROPHORESIS
ELECTROPHORESIS, PROTEIN; SEE PROTEIN ELECTROPHORESIS
ENA COMPLEX; SEE EXTRACTABLE NUCLEAR ANTIGEN

ENDOMYSIAL ANTIBODIES

Normal: not detected
Present in: celiac disease, dermatitis herpetiformis

EOSINOPHIL COUNT

Normal range: 1% to 4% eosinophils (0-440/mm^3)
Elevated in: allergy, parasitic infestations (trichinosis, aspergillosis, hydatidosis), angioneurotic edema, drug reactions, warfarin sensitivity, collagen-vascular diseases, acute hypereosinophilic syndrome, eosinophilic nonallergic rhinitis, myeloproliferative disorders, Hodgkin's lymphoma, non-Hodgkin's lymphoma (NHL), radiation therapy, L-tryptophan ingestion, urticaria, pernicious anemia, pemphigus, inflammatory bowel disease, bronchial asthma

EPINEPHRINE, PLASMA

Normal range: 0-90 pg/ml
Elevated in: pheochromocytomas, neuroblastomas, stress, vigorous exercise, ingestion of certain foods (bananas, chocolate, coffee, tea, vanilla), hypoglycemia

EPSTEIN-BARR VIRUS (EBV) SEROLOGY

Normal range: IgG anti-VCA <1:10 or negative
IgM anti-VCA <1:10 or negative
Anti-EBNA <1.5 or negative
Abnormal: IgG anti-VCA >1:10 or positive indicates either current or previous infection
IgM anti-VCA >1:10 or positive indicates current or recent infection
Anti-EBNA ≥1.5 or positive indicates previous infection
Figure 2-6 illustrates the pattern of EBV serology during acute infection.

ERYTHROCYTE SEDIMENTATION RATE (ESR) (WESTERGREN)

Normal range:
Male: 0-15 mm/hr
Female: 0-20 mm/hr
Elevated in: inflammatory states (acute-phase reactant), collagen-vascular diseases, infections, MI, neoplasms, hyperthyroidism, hypothyroidism, rouleaux formation, elderly, pregnancy

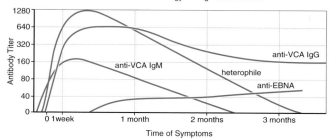

Figure 2-6 Patterns of Epstein-Barr virus serology during acute infection. (*From Young NS, Gerson SL, High KA, eds: Clinical Hematology, St. Louis, Mosby, 2006.*)

Note: Sedimentation rates greater than 100 mm/hr are strongly associated with serious underlying disease (collagen-vascular, infection, malignancy). Some clinicians use ESR as a "sickness index"; high rates encountered without obvious reason should be repeated rather than pursuing extensive search for occult disease.

Decreased in: sickle cell disease, polycythemia, corticosteroids, spherocytosis, anisocytosis, hypofibrinogenemia, increased serum viscosity, microcytosis

ERYTHROPOIETIN (EP)

Normal: 3.7-16.0 IU/L by radioimmunoassay

Erythropoietin is a glycoprotein secreted by the kidneys that stimulates RBC production by acting on erythroid committed stem cells.

Increased in: patients with severe anemia (generally extremely high; hematocrit [Hct] <25, hemoglobin [Hb] <7), such as in cases of aplastic anemia, severe hemolytic anemia, hematologic cancers. Very high in patients with mild to moderate anemia (Hct 25-35, Hb 7-10); high in patients with mild anemia (e.g., AIDS, myelodysplasia).

Erythropoietin can be inappropriately elevated in patients with malignant neoplasms, renal cysts, meningioma, hemingioblastoma, and leiomyoma and after renal transplant.

Decreased in: renal failure, polycythemia vera, autonomic neuropathy

ESTRADIOL (SERUM)

Normal range:
Male, adult: 10-50 pg/ml
Female, premenopausal: 30-400 pg/ml, depending on phase of menstrual cycle
Female, postmenopausal: 0-30 pg/ml
Decreased in: ovarian failure
Elevated in: tumors of ovary, testis, adrenal glands, or nonendocrine sites (rare)

ESTROGENS, TOTAL

Normal:
Male: 20-80 pg/ml
Female follicular phase: 60-200 pg/ml
Female luteal phase: 160-400 pg/ml
Female postmenopausal: <130 pg/ml
Elevated in: ovarian tumor producing estrogens, testicular tumors, tumors or hyperplasia of adrenal cortex, chorioepithelioma
Decreased in: menopause, primary ovarian failure, hypopituitarism, anorexia nervosa, gonadotropin-releasing hormone (GnRH) deficiency, psychogenic stress

ETHANOL (BLOOD)

Normal range:
negative (values <10 mg/dl are considered negative)
Ethanol is metabolized at 10-25 mg/dl/hr. Levels 80 mg/dl or higher are considered evidence of impairment for driving. Fatal blood concentration is considered to be more than 400 mg/dl.

EXTRACTABLE NUCLEAR ANTIGEN (ENA COMPLEX, ANTI-RNP ANTIBODY, ANTI-SM, ANTI-SMITH)

Normal: negative
Present in: SLE, rheumatoid arthritis, Sjögren's syndrome, mixed connective tissue disease (MCTD)

FDP; SEE FIBRIN DEGRADATION PRODUCT

FACTOR V LEIDEN

Test description: PCR test performed on whole blood or tissue. This single mutation, found in 2% to 8% in the general Caucasian population, is the single most common cause of hereditary thrombophilia.

FECAL FAT, QUALITATIVE; SEE SUDAN III STAIN

FECAL FAT, QUANTITATIVE (72-HOUR COLLECTION)

Normal range: 2-6 g/24 hr
Elevated in: malabsorption syndrome

FECAL GLOBIN IMMUNOCHEMICAL TEST

Normal: negative. This test is performed by immunochromatography on a cellulose strip that has been impregnated with various antibodies. The test uses a small amount of toilet water as the specimen and is placed onto absorbent pads of card similar to a traditional occult blood (OB) card. There is no direct handling of stool. This test is specific for the globin portion of the hemoglobin molecule, which confers lower GI bleeding specificity. It specifically detects blood from the lower GI tract, whereas guaiac tests are not lower GI specific. It is more sensitive than a typical Hemoccult test (detection limit 50 μg Hb/g feces versus > 500 μg Hb/g feces for Hemoccult). It has no dietary restrictions and gives no false positives due to plant peroxidases and red meats. It has no medication restrictions. Iron supplements and NSAIDs do not cause false positives. Vitamin C does not cause false negatives.

Positive in: lower GI bleeding

FERRITIN (SERUM)

Normal range: 18-300 ng/ml
Elevated in: inflammatory states, liver disease (ferritin elevated from necrotic hepatocytes), hyperthyroidism, neoplasms (neuroblastomas, lymphomas, leukemia, breast carcinoma), iron replacement therapy, hemochromatosis, hemosiderosis
Decreased in: iron deficiency anemia

FIBRIN DEGRADATION PRODUCT (FDP)

Normal range: <10 μg/ml
Elevated in: DIC, primary fibrinolysis, pulmonary embolism, severe liver disease
Note: The presence of rheumatoid factor may cause falsely elevated FDP.

FIBRINOGEN

Normal range: 200-400 mg/dl
Elevated in: tissue inflammation or damage (acute-phase protein reactant), oral contraceptive use, pregnancy, acute infection, MI
Decreased in: DIC, hereditary afibrinogenemia, liver disease, primary or secondary fibrinolysis, cachexia

FLUORESCENT TREPONEMAL ANTIBODY; SEE FTA-ABS

FOLATE (FOLIC ACID)

Normal range:
  Plasma: Low: <3.4 ng/ml
    Normal: >5.4 ng/ml
  RBC: >280 ng/ml

Decreased in: folic acid deficiency (inadequate intake, malabsorption), alcoholism, drug therapy (methotrexate, trimethoprim, phenytoin, oral contraceptives, azulfadine), vitamin B_{12} deficiency (defective red cell folate absorption), hemolytic anemia

Elevated in: folic acid therapy

FOLLICLE-STIMULATING HORMONE (FSH)

Normal range:
Male, adult <22 IU/L
Female adult, midcycle <40 IU/L
Female non-midcycle <20 IU/L
Female postmenopausal 40-160 IU/L

Elevated in: primary hypogonadism, gonadal failure, alcoholism, Klinefelter's syndrome, testicular feminization, anorchia, castration

Decreased in: precocious puberty related to adrenal tumors, congenital adrenal hyperplasia. Normal FSH in an adult nonovulating female is indicative of hypothalamic/pituitary dysfunction.

FREE T_4; SEE T_4, FREE
FREE THYROXINE INDEX

Normal range: 1.1-4.3

Serum free T_4 directly measures unbound thyroxine. Free T_4 can be measured by equilibrium dialysis (gold standard of free T_4 assays) or by immunometric techniques (influenced by serum levels of lipids, proteins, and certain drugs). The free thyroxine index (FTI) can also be easily calculated by multiplying T_4 times T_3RU and dividing the result by 100; the FTI corrects for any abnormal T_4 values secondary to protein binding:

$$FTI = T_4 \times T_3RU/100$$
Normal values equal 1.1 to 4.3

FSH; SEE FOLLICLE-STIMULATING HORMONE
FTA-ABS (SERUM)

Normal: nonreactive

Reactive in: syphilis, other treponemal diseases (yaws, pinta, bejel), SLE, pregnancy

FUROSEMIDE STIMULATION TEST

Normal: This test is performed by giving 60 mg furosemide orally after overnight fast. The patient should be on a normal diet without medications the week before the test. Normal results: renin 1-6 ng Al/ml/hr.

Elevated in: renovascular hypertension, Bartter's syndrome, high-renin essential hypertension, pheochromocytoma

No response in: primary aldosteronism, low-renin essential hypertension, hyporeninemic hypoaldosteronism

GAMMA-GLUTAMYL TRANSFERASE (GGT); SEE γ-GLUTAMYL TRANSFERASE
GASTRIN (SERUM)

Normal range: 0-180 pg/ml

Elevated in: Zollinger-Ellison syndrome (gastrinoma), use of proton pump inhibitors, chronic renal failure, gastric ulcer, chronic atrophic gastritis, pyloric obstruction, malignant neoplasms of the stomach, H_2 blockers, calcium therapy, ulcerative colitis, rheumatoid arthritis

GASTRIN STIMULATION TEST

Normal: Gastrin stimulation test after calcium infusion is performed by giving a calcium infusion (15 mg Ca/Kg in 500 ml normal saline over 4 hours). Serum is drawn in fasting state before infusion and at 1, 2, 3, and 4 hours. Normal response is little or no increase over baseline gastrin level.

Elevated in: gastrinoma (gastrin > 400 pg/ml), duodenal ulcer (gastrin level increase < 400 ng/L)

Decreased in: pernicious anemia, atrophic gastritis

GLIADIN ANTIBODIES, IgA and IgG

Normal: < 25 U, equivocal 20-25 U, positive > 25 U. This test is useful to monitor compliance with gluten-free diet in patients with celiac disease.

Elevated in: celiac disease with dietary noncompliance

GLOMERULAR BASEMENT MEMBRANE ANTIBODY

Normal: negative
Present in: Goodpasture's syndrome

GLOMERULAR FILTRATION RATE

Normal:
Age 20-29: 116 ml/min/1.73 m2
Age 30-39: 107 ml/min/1.73 m2
Age 40-49: 99 ml/min/1.73 m2
Age 50-59: 93 ml/min/1.73 m2
Age 60-69: 85 ml/min/1.73 m2
Age ≥ 70: 75 ml/min/1.73 m2
Decreased in: renal insufficiency, decrease renal blood flow

GLUCAGON

Normal: 20-100 pg/ml
Elevated in: glucagonoma (900-7800 pg/ml), chronic renal failure, diabetes mellitus, drug therapy (glucocorticoids, insulin, nifedipine, danazol, sympathomimetic amines)
Decreased in: hyperlipoproteinemia (types III, IV), beta blockers use, secretin therapy

GLUCOSE, FASTING

Normal range: 70-110 mg/dl
Elevated in: diabetes mellitus, stress, infections, MI, CVA, Cushing's syndrome, acromegaly, acute pancreatitis, glucagonoma, hemochromatosis, drug therapy (glucocorticoids, diuretics [thiazides, loop diuretics]), impaired glucose tolerance
Decreased in: prolonged fasting, excessive dose of insulin or hypoglycemic agents, insulinoma

GLUCOSE, POSTPRANDIAL

Normal range: <140 mg/dl
Elevated in: diabetes mellitus, impaired glucose tolerance
Decreased in: postgastrointestinal resection, reactive hypoglycemia, hereditary fructose intolerance, galactosemia, leucine sensitivity

GLUCOSE TOLERANCE TEST

Normal values above fasting:
30 minutes: 30-60 mg/dl

60 minutes: 20-50 mg/dl
120 minutes: 5-15 mg/dl
180 minutes: fasting level or below
Abnormal in: impaired glucose tolerance, diabetes mellitus, Cushing's syndrome, acromegaly, pheochromocytoma, gestational diabetes

GLUCOSE-6-PHOSPHATE DEHYDROGENASE (G_6PD) SCREEN (BLOOD)

Normal: G_6PD enzyme activity detected
Abnormal: If a deficiency is detected, quantitation of G_6PD is necessary; a G_6PD screen may be falsely interpreted as "normal" after an episode of hemolysis because most G_6PD deficient cells have been destroyed.

γ-GLUTAMYL TRANSFERASE (GGT)

Normal range: 0-30 U/L
Elevated in: chronic alcoholic liver disease, neoplasms (hepatoma, metastatic disease to the liver, carcinoma of the pancreas), nephrotic syndrome, sepsis, cholestasis, drug therapy (phenytoin, barbiturates)

GLYCATED (GLYCOSYLATED) HEMOGLOBIN (HbA_{lc})

Normal range: 4.0% to 6.0%
Note: HbA1c greater than 9% correlates with a mean glucose higher than 200 mg/dl. The goal of therapy should be an HbA1c less than 7%.
Elevated in: uncontrolled diabetes mellitus (glycated hemoglobin levels reflect the level of glucose control over the preceding 120 days), lead toxicity, alcoholism, iron deficiency anemia, hypertriglyceridemia
Decreased in: hemolytic anemias; decreased RBC survival; pregnancy, acute or chronic blood loss; chronic renal failure; insulinoma; congenital spherocytosis; Hb S, Hb C, Hb D diseases

GROWTH HORMONE

Normal:
Male: 1-9 ng/ml
Female: 1-16 ng/ml
Elevated in: pituitary gigantism, acromegaly, ectopic growth hormone (GH) secretion, cirrhosis, renal failure, anorexia nervosa, stress, exercise, prolonged fasting, drug therapy (amphetamines, beta blockers, insulin, levodopa, metoclopramide, clonidine, vasopressin)
Decreased in: hypopituitarism, pituitary dwarfism, adrenocortical hyperfunction, drug therapy (bromocriptine, corticosteroids, glucose)

GROWTH HORMONE–RELEASING HORMONE

Normal: <50 pg/ml
Elevated in: acromegaly caused by GHRH secretion by neoplasms

GROWTH HORMONE SUPPRESSION TEST (AFTER GLUCOSE)

Normal: This test is done by giving 1.75 g glucose/kg orally after overnight fast. Blood is drawn at baseline, after 60 minutes, and after 120 minutes of glucose load. Normal response is growth hormone suppression to less than 2 ng/ml or undetectable levels.
Abnormal: There is no or incomplete suppression from the high basal level in gigantism or acromegaly.

HAM TEST (ACID SERUM TEST)

Normal: negative

Positive in: paroxysmal nocturnal hemoglobinuria (PNH)

False-positive in: hereditary or acquired spherocytosis, recent transfusion with aged RBC, aplastic anemia, myeloproliferative syndromes, leukemia, hereditary dyserythropoietic anemia type II (HEMPAS)

HAPTOGLOBIN (SERUM)

Normal range: 50-220 mg/dl

Elevated in: inflammation (acute-phase reactant), collagen-vascular diseases, infections (acute-phase reactant), drug therapy (androgens), obstructive liver disease

Decreased in: hemolysis (intravascular more than extravascular), megaloblastic anemia, severe liver disease, large tissue hematomas, infectious mononucleosis, drug therapy (oral contraceptives)

HDL; SEE HIGH-DENSITY LIPOPROTEIN CHOLESTEROL

HELICOBACTER PYLORI (SEROLOGY, STOOL ANTIGEN)

Normal range: not detected

Detected in: *H. pylori* infection. Positive serology can indicate current or past infection. Positive stool antigen test indicates acute infection (sensitivity and specificity >90%). Stool testing should be delayed at least 2 weeks after eradication therapy.

Table 2-2 describes diagnostic tests for *H. pylori.*

HEMATOCRIT

Normal range:

Male: 39% to 49%

Female: 33% to 43%

Elevated in: polycythemia vera, smoking, COPD, high altitudes, dehydration, hypovolemia

Decreased in: blood loss (GI, genitourinary [GU]), anemia, pregnancy, prolonged medical illness, renal failure

HEMOGLOBIN

Normal range:

Male: 13.6-17.7 g/dl

Female: 12.0-15.0 g/dl

Elevated in: hemoconcentration, dehydration, polycythemia vera, COPD, high altitudes, false elevations (hyperlipemic plasma, WBCs $> 50,000$ mm^3), stress

Decreased in: hemorrhage (GI, GU), anemia, prolonged medical illness, renal failure

HEMOGLOBIN ELECTROPHORESIS

Normal range:

HbA$_1$: 95% to 98%

HbA$_2$: 1.5% to 3.5%

HbF: <2%

HbC: absent

HbS: absent

HEMOGLOBIN, GLYCATED; SEE GLYCATED HEMOGLOBIN

HEMOGLOBIN, GLYCOSYLATED; SEE GLYCATED HEMOGLOBIN

HEMOGLOBIN H

Normal: negative

Present in: hemoglobin H disease, alpha thalassemia trait, unstable hemoglobin disorders

TABLE 2-2 Diagnostic Tests for *H. pylori**

Methods	Advantages	Disadvantages	Usefulness
Noninvasive			
Serology	Noninvasive, relatively cheap	Requires validation in local patient	Initial diagnosis, no follow-up after therapy
^{14}C urea breath test	Rapid, allows distinction between current and past infection	Involves ingestion of radioactivity. Reduced sensitivity with acid suppression or antibiotics	Initial diagnosis, follow-up of treatment regimens
^{14}C urea breath test	No radioactivity, as for ^{14}C	Complex equipment, expensive. Reduced sensitivity with acid suppression or antibiotics	Initial diagnosis, follow-up of treatment regimens
Invasive			
Rapid urease test	Rapid, inexpensive	Invasive. Reduced sensitivity in those on acid suppression or with recent or active bleeding	Initial diagnosis
Histology	Allows assessment of mucosa	Invasive, costly	Assess gastritis, metaplasia, atrophy, etc., initial diagnosis
Culture	Specificity: 100%	Invasive, costly, slow, less sensitive	Initial diagnosis, antimicrobial sensitivities, strain typing (macrolide resistance 4%-12%); metronidazole resistance is common

*Testing should only be performed if treatment is planned.
From Talley NJ, Martin CJ: *Clinical Gastroenterology*, ed 2, Sidney, Churchill Livingstone, 2006.

HEMOGLOBIN, URINE; SEE URINE HEMOGLOBIN
HEMOSIDERIN, URINE; SEE URINE HEMOSIDERIN
HEPARIN-INDUCED THROMBOCYTOPENIA ANTIBODIES
Normal: antigen assay: negative < 0.45, weak 0.45-1.0, strong > 1.0
Elevated in: heparin-induced thrombocytopenia

HEPATITIS A ANTIBODY
Normal: negative
Present in: viral hepatitis A; can be IgM or IgG (if IgM, acute hepatitis A; if IgG, previous infection with hepatitis A)

HEPATITIS B CORE ANTIBODY

Normal: negative

Present in: hepatitis B. Anti-HBc assay is the first antibody test to become positive with exposure to hepatitis B virus (HBV) and persists the longest after resolution of acute infection.

Figure 2-7 describes viral antigens and antibodies in hepatitis B infection

HEPATITIS B DNA

Normal: negative

Present in: active hepatitis B infection. It implies infectivity of the serum. This test is currently used to assess the response of hepatitis B to therapy.

HEPATITIS B e ANTIGEN AND ANTIBODY

Normal: negative. These tests are ordered together and should only be used in patients who are chronically HBsAg positive. The main utility of these tests is to assess response of hepatitis B infection to therapy.

Present: The presence of HBeAg implies that infective hepatitis B virus is present in serum. However, its absence on conversion to anti-HBe does not rule out infection, especially in persons infected with genotypes other than A. Measurement of HBV-DNA is useful in persons with increased alanine aminotransferase (ALT) but negative HBeAg.

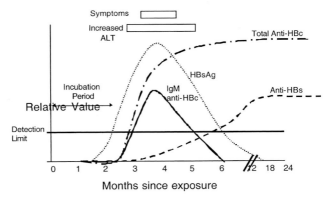

Figure 2-7 Typical time course for appearance of viral antigens and antiviral antibodies in acute hepatitis B (HBV) infection. After an incubation period of 1 to 3 months, surface antigen (HBsAg) is the first viral marker to appear. During the incubation period and while no detectable antibody is present, the patient remains asymptomatic. After 3 to 6 months total, antibody to the core antigen (anti-HBc) appears, typically first as an IgM antibody (IgM anti-HBc). At the time of antibody development, symptoms of acute infection begin, accompanied by increased cytoplasmic enzymes and, in many cases, by jaundice. At the time of development of jaundice, most patients still have measurable HBsAg. In a few patients, neither surface antigen nor its antibody is detectable, leaving IgM anti-HBc as the only marker of acute infection ("core window"). Development of anti-HBc indicates clearance of infectious virus and recovery from infection. IgM anti-HBc persists for about 3 to 6 months, but total anti-HBc is typically present for life. *(From Henry JB, ed: Clinical Diagnosis and Management by Laboratory Methods, Philadelphia, WB Saunders, 2001.)*

HEPATITIS B SURFACE ANTIBODY

Normal: negative
Present: after vaccination for hepatitis B (a level >10 U/L for postvaccine testing is the accepted concentration that indicates protection), after infection with hepatitis B (it generally appears several weeks after disappearance of HBsAg).

HEPATITIS B SURFACE ANTIGEN (HBsAg)

Normal: not detected
Detected in: acute viral hepatitis type B, chronic hepatitis B

HEPATITIS C ANTIBODY (ANTI-HCV)

Normal: negative
Present in: hepatitis C. Centers for Disease Control and Prevention (CDC) guidelines recommend confirmation with recombinant immunoblot assay (RIBA) before reporting anti-HCV as positive. HCV-RNA can also be obtained if there is a high clinical suspicion of HCV despite a negative anti-HVC, especially in immunosuppressed individuals or in the setting of acute hepatitis. Anti-HCV and the RIBA often do not become positive during an acute infection; thus repeat testing several months later is required if HCV-RNA is negative.
   Figure 2-8 describes antibody and antigen patterns in hepatitis C infection.

HEPATITIS C RNA

Normal: negative
Elevated in: hepatitis C. Detection of hepatitis C RNA is used to confirm current infection and to monitor treatment. Quantitative assays (viral load) are needed before treatment to assess response (<2 log decrease after 12-week treatment indicates lack of response).

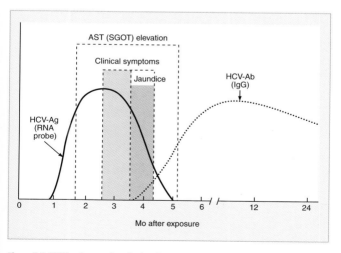

Figure 2-8 HCV antigen and antibody. *(From Ravel R: Clinical Laboratory Medicine, ed 6, St. Louis, Mosby, 1995.)*

HEPATITIS D ANTIGEN AND ANTIBODY

Normal: negative

Elevated in: hepatitis D. Hepatitis D is a replication-defective RNA virus that requires the surface coat of hepatitis B (HBsAg) to become an infectious virus. Testing for hepatitis D is therefore done only in patients positive for HBsAg. It is useful in patients with chronic hepatitis B if there is an exacerbation of stable hepatitis.

Her-2/nue

Normal: negative

Present in: 25% to 30% of primary breast cancers. It can also be found in other epithelial tumors, including lung, hepatocellular, pancreatic, colon, stomach, ovarian, cervical, and bladder cancers. Trastuzumab (Herceptin) is a humanized monoclonal antibody against Her-2/nue. Test is useful to identify patients with metastatic, recurrent, or treatment-refractory unresectable locally advanced breast cancer for trastuzumab treatment.

HERPES SIMPLEX VIRUS (HSV)

Test description: PCR test can be performed on serum biopsy samples, CSF, vitreous humor

Table 2-3 describes laboratory diagnosis of herpes virus infections.

HETEROPHIL ANTIBODY

Normal: negative

Positive in: infectious mononucleosis

HFE SCREEN FOR HEREDITARY HEMOCHROMATOSIS

Test description: PCR test can be performed on whole blood or tissue. One mutation (C282Y) and two polymorphisms (H63D, S65C) account for the majority of alleles associated with this disease.

HIGH-DENSITY LIPOPROTEIN (HDL) CHOLESTEROL

Normal range:

Male: 45-70 mg/dl

Female: 50-90 mg/dl

Increased in: use of fenofibrate, gemfibrozil, nicotinic acid, estrogens; regular aerobic exercise; mild to moderate (1 oz) daily alcohol intake, omega-3-fatty acids

Decreased in: familial deficiency of apoproteins, liver disease, probucol ingestion, sedentary lifestyle, acute MI, CVA, starvation

Note: A cholesterol/HDL ratio 4.5 or more is associated with increased risk of coronary artery disease.

Figure 2-9 describes the composition of the major classes of lipoproteins.

HOMOCYSTEINE, PLASMA

Normal range:

0-30 years: 4.6-8.1 micromol/L

30-59 years:

Males: 6.3-11.2 micromol/L

Females: 4-5-7.9 micromol/L

>59 years: 5.8-11.9 micromol/L

Increased: thrombophilic states; B_6, B_{12}, folic acid, riboflavin deficiency; pregnancy; homocystinuria

Note: An increased homocysteine level is an independent risk factor for atherosclerosis.

TABLE 2-3 Laboratory Diagnosis of Herpes Virus Infections

Virus	Disease Manifestation	Virus Culture	Serology	Antigen Detection	DNA Amplification
HSV-1	Skin lesions	+ + +	+ +	+	+ + +
	CNS infection	−	+	−	+ + +
HSV-2	Genital lesions	+ + +	+	+	+ + +
	CNS infection	−	+	−	+ + +
VZV	Skin lesions	+ +	+	+ +	+ + +
	CNS infection	−	+ +	−	+ + +
CMV	Mononucleosis-like illness	−	+ + +	−	−
	Neonatal disease	+ + +	+ +	−	+ + +
	Systemic infection in immunocompromised	+	+	+ +	+ + +
	CNS disease	−	+	−	+ + +
EBV	Mononucleosis-like illness	−	+ + +	−	−
	Systemic infection in immunocompromised	−	+	+	+ + +
	CNS disease	−	+	−	+ + +
HHV-6	Exanthema subitum	+	+ + +	−	−
	CNS disease	−	+ +	−	+ + +
HHV-8	Kaposi's sarcoma	−	+	−	+ + +

HHV, Human herpesvirus; VZV, varicella zoster virus.
From Cohen J, Powderly WG: *Infectious Diseases,* ed 2, St. Louis, Mosby, 2004.

Composition of the major classes of lipoproteins

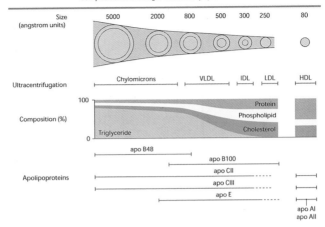

Figure 2-9 Composition of the major classes of lipoproteins. Although each of the lipoproteins is distinct with respect to its relative proportions of cholesterol, triglycerides, phospholipids, and apolipoproteins, considerable heterogeneity exists within each lipoprotein class. Lipoproteins are graded according to their density: very low (VLDL), low (LDL), intermediate (IDL), or high (HDL). Clinical measures of LDL include both LDL and IDL. *(From Besser CM, Thorner MO: Comprehensive Clinical Endocrinology, ed 3, St. Louis, Mosby, 2002.)*

Hs-CRP; SEE C-REACTIVE PROTEIN
HSV; SEE HERPES SIMPLEX VIRUS
HUMAN HERPES VIRUS 8 (HHV8)

Test description: PCR test can be performed on whole blood, tissue, bone marrow, and urine. HHV8 is found in all forms of Kaposi's sarcoma.

HUMAN IMMUNODEFICIENCY VIRUS ANTIBODY, TYPE 1 (HIV-1)

Normal range: not detected

Abnormal result: HIV antibodies usually appear in the blood 1 to 4 months after infection.

Testing sequence:

1. ELISA is the recommended initial screening test. Sensitivity and specificity is greater than 99%. False-positive ELISA may occur with autoimmune disorders, administration of immune globulin manufactured before 1985 within 6 weeks of testing, presence of rheumatoid factor, presence of DLA-DR antibodies in multigravida females, administration of influenza vaccine within 3 months of testing, hemodialysis, positive plasma reagin test, and certain medical disorders (hemophilia, hypergammaglobulinemia, alcoholic hepatitis).

2. A positive ELISA is confirmed with Western blot (Figure 2-10). False-positive Western blot may be caused by connective tissue disorders, human leukocyte antigen (HLA) antibodies, polyclonal gammopathies, hyperbilirubinemia, presence of antibody to another human retrovirus, or cross-reaction with other

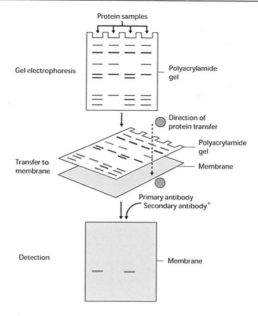

Figure 2-10 Western blot technique. The solubilized protein mix is separated on a polyacrylamide gel and transferred electrophoretically to a membrane. The membrane is soaked in a buffer containing antibody. The bound antibody is detected by a chromogenic or chemiluminescent assay. *(From Bolognia JL, Jorizzo JL, Rapini RP: Dermatology, St. Louis, Mosby, 2003.)*

non–virus-derived proteins in healthy persons. Undetermined Western blot may occur in AIDS patients with advanced immunodeficiency (from loss of antibodies) and in recent HIV infections.

3. PCR is used to confirm indeterminate Western blot results or negative results in persons with suspected HIV infection.

Figure 2-11 illustrates the immune response to HIV and relationship to clinical symptoms.

5-HYDROXYINDOLE-ACETIC ACID, URINE; SEE URINE 5-HYDROXYINDOLE-ACETIC ACID

HUMAN PAPILLOMA VIRUS (HPV)

Test description: PCR test can be performed on cervical smears, biopsies, scrapings, liquid cytology specimen, and anogenital tissues.

HUNTINGTON'S DISEASE PCR

Test description: PCR test can be performed on whole blood. Huntington's disease is caused by the expansion of the trinucleotide repeat CAG within IT 15 (huntingtion).

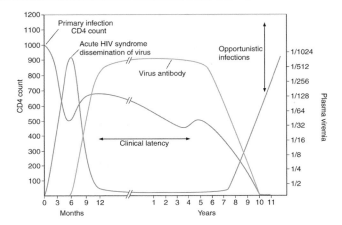

Figure 2-11 Immune response to HIV and relationship to clinical symptomatology and development of AIDS. After primary HIV infection, there is a period of viremia followed by development of IgM and the IgG antibody 4 to 7 weeks later. Development of antibody is accompanied by disappearance of the virus from the circulation. Eventually CD4 counts decrease, viral antibody titers decline, and viremia recurs. *(From Young NS, Gerson SL, High KA, eds: Clinical Hematology, St. Louis, Mosby, 2006.)*

IMMUNE COMPLEX ASSAY

Normal: negative
Detected in: collagen-vascular disorders, glomerulonephritis, neoplastic diseases, malaria, primary biliary cirrhosis, chronic acute hepatitis, bacterial endocarditis, vasculitis

IMMUNOGLOBULINS

Normal range:
 IgA: 50-350 mg/dl
 IgD: <6 mg/dl
 IgE: <25 μg/dl
 IgG: 800-1500 mg/dl
 IgM: 45-150 mg/dl
 Elevated in: IgA: lymphoproliferative disorders, Berger's nephropathy, chronic infections, autoimmune disorders, liver disease
 IgE: allergic disorders, parasitic infections, immunologic disorders, IgE myeloma, AIDS, pemphigoid
 IgG: chronic granulomatous infections, infectious diseases, inflammation, myeloma, liver disease
 IgM: primary biliary cirrhosis, infectious diseases (brucellosis, malaria), Waldenström's macroglobulinemia, liver disease
 Decreased in: IgA: nephrotic syndrome, protein-losing enteropathy, congenital deficiency, lymphocytic leukemia, ataxia-telangiectasia, chronic sinopulmonary disease
 IgE: hypogammaglobulinemia, neoplasm (breast, bronchial, cervical), ataxia-telangiectasia
 IgG: congenital or acquired deficiency, lymphocytic leukemia, phenytoin, methylprednisolone, nephrotic syndrome, protein-losing enteropathy

IgM: congenital deficiency, lymphocytic leukemia, nephrotic syndrome

INFLUENZA A AND B TESTS
Test description: PCR can be performed on nasopharyngeal swab, wash, or aspirate.

INR; SEE INTERNATIONAL NORMALIZED RATIO
INSULIN AUTOANTIBODIES
Normal: negative

Present in: exogenous insulin from insulin therapy. The presence of islet cell antibodies indicates ongoing beta cell destruction. This test is useful in the early diagnosis of type 1a diabetes mellitus and in the identification of patients at high risk for type 1a diabetes.

INSULIN, FREE
Normal: <17 microU/ml

Elevated in: insulin overdose, insulin resistance syndromes, endogenous hyperinsulinemia

Decreased in: inadequately treated type 1 DM

INSULIN-LIKE GROWTH FACTOR-1 (IGF-1), SERUM

Normal range:
Age 16-24: 182-780 ng/ml
Age 25-39: 114-492 ng/ml
Age 40-54: 90-360 ng/ml
Age > 55: 71-290 ng/ml

Elevated in: adolescence, acromegaly, pregnancy, precocious puberty, obesity

Decreased in: malnutrition, delayed puberty, diabetes mellitus, hypopituitarism, cirrhosis, old age

INSULIN-LIKE GROWTH FACTOR II
Normal: 288-736 ng/ml

Elevated in: hypoglycemia associated with non–islet cell tumors, hepatoma, and Wilms' tumor

Decreased in: growth hormone deficiency

INTERNATIONAL NORMALIZED RATIO (INR)
The INR is a comparative rating of prothrombin time (PT) ratios. The INR represents the observed PT ratio adjusted by the International Reference Sensitivity Index: INR = PT patient/PT mean. The INR provides a universal result indicative of what the patient's PT result would have been if measured by using the primary World Health Organization International Reference reagent. For proper interpretation of INR values, the patient should be on stable anticoagulant therapy. Normal range of INR is 0.8 to 1.2.

Recommended INR ranges:

Disorder	INR Range
Proximal deep vein thrombosis	2-3
Pulmonary embolism	2-3
Transient ischemic attacks	2-3
Atrial fibrillation	2-3
Mechanical prosthetic valves	3-4.5
Recurrent venous thromboembolic disease	3-4.5

INTRINSIC FACTOR ANTIBODIES

Normal: negative

Present in: pernicious anemia (>50% of patients). Cyanocobalamin may give false positive results.

IRON, SERUM

Normal: Male: 65-175 μg/dl; female: 50-1170 μg/dl

Elevated in: hemochromatosis, excessive iron therapy, repeated transfusions, lead poisoning, hemolytic anemia, aplastic anemia, pernicious anemia

Decreased in: iron deficiency anemia, hypothyroidism, chronic infection, pregnancy uremia

IRON-BINDING CAPACITY (Total Iron Binding Capacity [TIBC])

Normal range: 250-460 μg/dl

Elevated in: iron deficiency anemia, pregnancy, polycythemia, hepatitis, weight loss

Decreased in: anemia of chronic disease, hemochromatosis, chronic liver disease, hemolytic anemias, malnutrition (protein depletion)

IRON SATURATION (% TRANSFERRIN SATURATION)

Normal:

Male: 20% to 50%

Female: 15% to 50%

Elevated in: hemochromatosis, excessive iron intake, aplastic anemia, thalassemia, vitamin B_6 deficiency

Decreased in: hypochromic anemias, GI malignancy

LACTATE (BLOOD)

Normal range: 0.5-2.0 mEq/L

Elevated in: tissue hypoxia (shock, respiratory failure, severe CHF, severe anemia, carbon monoxide or cyanide poisononing), systemic disorders (liver or renal failure, seizures), abnormal intestinal flora (D-lactic acidosis), drugs or toxins (salicylates, ethanol, methanol, ethylene glycol), G6PD deficiency

LACTATE DEHYDROGENASE (LDH)

Normal range: 50-150 U/L

Elevated in: infarction of myocardium, lung, kidney; diseases of cardiopulmonary system, liver, collagen, CNS; hemolytic anemias, megaloblastic anemias, transfusions, seizures, muscle trauma, muscular dystrophy, acute pancreatitis, hypotension, shock, infectious mononucleosis, inflammation, neoplasia, intestinal obstruction, hypothyroidism

LACTATE DEHYDROGENASE ISOENZYMES

Normal range:

LDH_1: 22% to 36% (cardiac, RBCs)

LDH_2: 35% to 46% (cardiac, RBCs)

LDH_3: 13% to 26% (pulmonary)

LDH_4: 3% to 10% (striated muscle, liver)

LDH_5: 2% to 9% (striated muscle, liver)

Normal range:

$LDH_1 < LDH_2$

$LDH_5 < LDH_4$

Abnormal values:

$LDH_1 > LDH_2$:

MI (can also be seen with hemolytic anemias, pernicious anemia, folate deficiency, renal infarct)

$LDH_5 > LDH_4$: liver disease (cirrhosis, hepatitis, hepatic congestion)

LACTOSE TOLERANCE TEST (SERUM)
Normal: This test is performed by giving 2g/kg body weight lactose orally and drawing glucose level at 0, 30, 45, 60, and 90 minutes. A normal response is a change in glucose from fasting value to more than 30 mg/dl. An inconclusive response is an increase of 20 to 30 mg/dl; an abnormal response is an increase less than 20 mg/dl.
Abnormal in: lactase deficiency

LANOXIN; SEE DIGOXIN
LAP SCORE; SEE LEUKOCYTE ALKALINE PHOSPHATASE
LEAD

Normal:
Child: <10 µg/dl
Adult: <25 µg/dl; acceptable for industrial exposure <50 µg/dl
Elevated in: lead exposure, lead poisoning

LDH; SEE LACTATE DEHYDROGENASE
LDL; SEE LOW-DENSITY LIPOPROTEIN CHOLESTEROL
LEGIONELLA PNEUMOPHILA PCR
Test description: PCR can be performed on lung tissue, water sputum, bronchoalveolar lavage, and other respiratory fluids.

LEGIONELLA TITER
Normal: negative
Positive in: Legionnaire's disease (presumptive: ≥1:256 titer; definitive: fourfold titer increase to ≥1:128)

LEUKOCYTE ALKALINE PHOSPHATASE (LAP)
Normal range: 13-100
Elevated in: leukemoid reactions, neutrophilia resulting from infections (except in sickle cell crisis—no significant increase in LAP score), Hodgkin's disease, polycythemia vera, hairy cell leukemia, aplastic anemia, Down syndrome, myelofibrosis
Decreased in: acute and chronic granulocytic leukemia, thrombocytopenic purpura, paroxysmal nocturnal hemoglobinuria (PNH), hypophosphatemia, collagen disorders

LH; SEE LUTEINIZING HORMONE
LIPASE
Normal range: 0-160 U/L
Elevated in: acute pancreatitis, perforated peptic ulcer, carcinoma of pancreas (early stage), pancreatic duct obstruction, bowel infarction, intestinal obstruction

LIPOPROTEIN (A)
Normal:
Male: 1.35-19.6 mg/dl
Female: 1.24-20.1 mg/dl

Elevated in: coronary artery disease, uncontrolled diabetes, hypothyroidism, chronic renal failure, pregnancy, tobacco use, infections, nephritic syndrome

Decreased in: niacin, estrogens, tamoxifen therapy; omega-3 fatty acid use

LIPOPROTEIN CHOLESTEROL, LOW DENSITY; SEE LOW-DENSITY LIPOPROTEIN CHOLESTEROL

LIPOPROTEIN CHOLESTEROL, HIGH DENSITY; SEE HIGH-DENSITY LIPOPROTEIN CHOLESTEROL

LIVER KIDNEY MICROSOME TYPE 1 ANTIBODIES (LKM1)

Normal: <20 U

Elevated in: autoimmune hepatitis type 2

LOW-DENSITY LIPOPROTEIN (LDL) CHOLESTEROL

Normal range: <130 mg/dl (<70 mg/dl in diabetics and patients with cardiovascular risk factors)

Elevated in: diet high in saturated fat, familial hyperlipidemia, sedentary lifestyle, poorly controlled diabetes mellitus, nephritic syndrome, hypothyroidism

Decreased in: use of lipid-lowering agents (statins, niacin, ezetimibe, cholestyramine, colesevelam), starvation, malabsorption, abetalipoproteinemia, hyperthyroidism, hepatic failure, carcinoma, infection, inflammation

LUPUS ANTICOAGULANT (LA) TEST

Normal: negative

Present in: antiphospholipid antibody syndrome. False positives may occur with oral anticoagulant therapy, factor deficiency, and specific factor inhibitors.

LUTEINIZING HORMONE (LH), BLOOD

Normal range:

Female, adult: Follicular phase: 1.0-18.0 IU/L

  Midcycle phase: 20.0-80.0 IU/L

  Luteal phase: 0.5-18.0 IU/L

  Postmenopausal: 12.0-55.0 IU/L

Male, adult: 1.0-9.0 IU/L

Elevated in: gonadal failure, anorchia, menopause, testicular feminization syndrome

Decreased in: primary pituitary or hypothalamic failure

LYMPHOCYTES

Normal range: 15% to 40%:

  Total lymphocyte count: 800-2600/mm^3

  Total T-lymphocytes: 800-2200/mm^3

  CD4 lymphocytes $\geq$ 400/mm^3

  CD8 lymphocytes = 200-800/mm^3

  Normal CD4/CD8 ratio is 2.0

Elevated in: chronic infections, infectious mononucleosis and other viral infections, CLL, Hodgkin's disease, ulcerative colitis, hypoadrenalism, ITP

Decreased in: HIV infection, bone marrow suppression from chemotherapeutic agents or chemotherapy, aplastic anemia, neoplasms, steroids, adrenocortical hyperfunction, neurologic disorders (multiple sclerosis, myasthenia gravis, Guillain-Barré syndrome)

CD4 lymphocytes are calculated as total WBCs $\times$ % lymphocytes $\times$ % lymphocytes stained with CD4. They are decreased in AIDS and other forms of immune dysfunction.

MAGNESIUM (SERUM)

Normal range: 1.8-3.0 mg/dl

Elevated in:
a. Renal failure (decreased GFR)
b. Decreased renal excretion secondary to salt depletion
c. Abuse of antacids and laxatives containing magnesium in patients with renal insufficiency
d. Endocrinopathies (deficiency of mineralocorticoid or thyroid hormone)
e. Increased tissue breakdown (rhabdomyolysis)
f. Redistribution: acute DKA, pheochromocytoma
g. Other: lithium therapy, volume depletion, familial hypocalciuric hypercalcemia

Decreased in:
a. GI and nutritional
  1. Defective GI absorption (malabsorption)
  2. Inadequate dietary intake (e.g., alcoholics)
  3. Parenteral therapy without magnesium
  4. Chronic diarrhea, villous adenoma, prolonged nasogastric suction, fistulas (small bowel, biliary)
b. Excessive renal losses
  1. Diuretic use
  2. Renal tubular acidosis (RTA)
  3. Diuretic phase of acute tubular necrosis (ATN)
  4. Endocrine disturbances (DKA, hyperaldosteronism, hyperthyroidism, hyperparathyroidism), SIADH, Bartter's syndrome, hypercalciuria, hypokalemia
  5. Cisplatin therapy; alcohol use; cyclosporine, digoxin, pentamidine, mannitol, amphotericin B, foscarnet, methotrexate therapy
  6. Antibiotic therapy (gentamicin, ticarcillin, carbenicillin)
  7. Redistribution: hypoalbuminemia, cirrhosis, administration of insulin and glucose, theophylline use, epinephrine use, acute pancreatitis, cardiopulmonary bypass
  8. Miscellaneous: sweating, burns, prolonged exercise, lactation, "hungry-bones" syndrome

MEAN CORPUSCULAR VOLUME (MCV)

Normal range: 76-100 μm^3

Elevated in: alcohol abuse, reticulocytosis, vitamin B_{12} deficiency, folic acid deficiency, liver disease, hypothyroidism, marrow aplasia, myelofibrosis

Decreased in: iron deficiency, anemia of chronic disease, thalassemia trait or syndrome, other hemoglobinopathies, sideroblastic anemia, chronic renal failure, lead poisoning

METANEPHRINES, URINE; SEE URINE METANEPHRINES

METHYLMALONIC ACID, SERUM

Normal: <0.2 micromol/L

Elevated in: Vitamin B_{12} deficiency, pregnancy, methylmalonic acidemia

MITOCHONDRIAL ANTIBODY (AMA)

Normal: negative

Present in: primary biliary cirrhosis (>90% of patients)

MONOCYTE COUNT

Normal range: 2% to 8%

Elevated in: viral diseases, parasites, infections, neoplasms, inflammatory bowel disease, monocytic leukemia, lymphomas, myeloma, sarcoidosis

Decreased in: viral syndrome, glucocorticoid administration, aplastic anemia, lymphocytic leukemia

MYCOPLASMA PNEUMONIAE PCR

Test description: PCR can be performed on sputum, bronchoalveolar lavage, nasopharyngeal and throat swabs, other respiratory fluids, and lung tissue

MYELIN BASIC PROTEIN, CEREBROSPINAL FLUID

Normal: <2.5 ng/ml

Elevated in: multiple sclerosis, CNS trauma, stroke, encephalitis

MYOGLOBIN, URINE; SEE URINE MYOGLOBIN
NATRIURETIC PEPTIDE; SEE B-TYPE NATRIURETIC PEPTIDE
NEISSERIA GONORRHOEAE PCR

Test description: Test can be performed on endocervical swab, urine, and intraurethral swab

NEUTROPHIL COUNT

Normal range: 50% to 70%

Subsets: Bands (early mature neutrophils): 2% to 6%
  Segs (mature neutrophils): 60% to 70%

Elevated in: acute bacterial infections, acute MI, stress, neoplasms, myelocytic leukemia

Decreased in: viral infections, aplastic anemias, immunosuppressive drugs, radiation therapy to bone marrow, agranulocytosis, drug therapy (antibiotics, antithyroidals), lymphocytic and monocytic leukemias

NOREPINEPHRINE

Normal range: 0-600 pg/ml

Elevated in: pheochromocytomas, neuroblastomas, stress, vigorous exercise, certain foods (bananas, chocolate, coffee, tea, vanilla)

5′ NUCLEOTIDASE

Normal range: 2-16 IU/L

Elevated in: biliary obstruction, metastatic neoplasms to liver, primary biliary cirrhosis, renal failure, pancreatic carcinoma, chronic active hepatitis

OSMOLALITY, SERUM

Normal range: 280-300 mOsm/kg

It can also be estimated by the following formula: $2([Na] + [K]) + Glucose/18 + BUN/2.8$.

Elevated in: dehydration, hypernatremia, diabetes insipidus, uremia, hyperglycemia, mannitol therapy, ingestion of toxins (ethylene glycol, methanol, ethanol), hypercalcemia, diuretic use

Decreased in: SIADH, hyponatremia, overhydration, Addison's disease, hypothyroidism

OSMOLALITY, URINE; SEE URINE OSMOLALITY
OSMOTIC FRAGILITY TEST

Normal: Hemolysis begins at 0.50, w/v (5.0 g/L) and is complete at 0.30, w/v (3.0 g/L) NaCl.

Elevated in: hereditary spherocytosis, hereditary stomatocytosis, spherocytosis associated with acquired immune hemolytic anemia

Decreased in: iron deficiency anemia, thalassemias, liver disease, leptocytosis associated with asplenia

PARACENTESIS FLUID

Testing and evaluation of results:
1. Process the fluid as follows:
   a. Tube 1: LDH, glucose, albumin
   b. Tube 2: protein, specific gravity
   c. Tube 3: cell count and differential
   d. Tube 4: save until further notice
2. Draw serum LDH, protein, albumin.
3. Gram stain, acid fast bacteria (AFB) stain, bacterial and fungal cultures, amylase, and triglycerides should be ordered only when clearly indicated; bedside inoculation of blood-culture bottles with ascitic fluid improves sensitivity in detecting bacterial growth.
4. If malignant ascites is suspected, consider a carcinoembryonic antigen level on the paracentesis fluid and cytologic evaluation.
5. In suspected spontaneous bacterial peritonitis (SBP) the incidence of positive cultures can be increased by injecting 10 to 20 ml of ascitic fluid into blood culture bottles.
6. Peritoneal effusion can be subdivided as exudative or transudative based on its characteristics.
7. The serum-ascites albumin gradient (serum albumin level–ascitic fluid albumin level) correlates directly with portal pressure and can also be used to classify ascites. Patients with gradients 1.1 g/dl or more have portal hypertension, and those with gradients less than 1.1 g/dl do not; the accuracy of this method is greater than 95%.
8. An ascitic fluid polymorphonuclear leukocyte count greater than 500/μl is suggestive of SBP.
9. A blood-ascitic fluid albumin gradient less than 1.1 g/dl is suggestive of malignant ascites.

Table 2-4 describes characteristics of paracentesis fluid in various disorders.

PARATHYROID HORMONE

Normal: Serum, intact molecule: 10-65 pg/ml; plasma 1.0-5.0 pmol/L

Elevated in: hyperparathyroidism (primary or secondary), pseudohypoparathyroidism, drug therapy (anticonvulsants, corticosteroids, lithium, INH, rifampin, phosphates), Zollinger-Ellison (ZE) syndrome, hereditary vitamin D deficiency

Decreased in: hypoparathyroidism, sarcoidosis, drug therapy (cimetidine, beta blockers), hyperthyroidism, hypomagnesemia

PARIETAL CELL ANTIBODIES

Normal: negative

Present in: pernicious anemia (> 90%), atrophic gastritis (up to 50%), thyroiditis (30%), Addison's disease, myasthenia gravis, Sjögren's syndrome, type 1 DM

PARTIAL THROMBOPLASTIN TIME (PTT), ACTIVATED THROMBOPLASTIN TIME (aPTT)

Normal range: 25-41 seconds

Elevated in: heparin therapy, coagulation factor deficiency (I, II, V, VIII, IX, X, XI, XII), liver disease, vitamin K deficiency, DIC, circulating anticoagulant, warfarin therapy, specific factor inhibition (PCN reaction, rheumatoid arthritis), thrombolytic therapy, nephrotic syndrome

TABLE 2-4 Characteristics of Paracentesis Fluid

Aetiology	Color	SAAG (g/L)	RBC (10⁶/L)	WBC (10⁶/L)	Cytology	Other
Cirrhosis	Straw	≥ 11	Few	< 250	—	—
Infected ascites	Straw	≥ 11	Few	≥ 250 polymorphs or ≥ 500 cells	—	+ culture
Neoplastic	Straw/haemorrhagic/mucinous	< 11	Variable	Variable	Malignant cells	—
Tuberulosis	Clear/turbid/ haemorrhagic	< 11	Many	> 1000 70% lymphocytes	—	Acid-fast bacilli + culture
Cardiac failure	Straw	≥ 11	0	< 250	—	—
Pancreatic	Turbid/ haemorrhagic	< 11	Variable	Variable	—	Amylase increased
Lymphatic obstruction or disruption	White	< 11	0	0	—	Fat globules on staining

SAAG, Serum ascites albumin gradient.
From Talley NJ, Martin CJ: *Clinical Gastroenterology*, ed 2, Sidney, Churchill Livingstone, 2006.

Note: This test is useful to evaluate the intrinsic coagulation system.

PEPSINOGEN I
Normal: 124-142 ng/ml
Elevated in: ZE syndrome, duodenal ulcer, acute gastritis
Decreased in: atrophic gastritis, gastric carcinoma, myxedema, pernicious anemia, Addison's disease

PFA: SEE PLATELET FUNCTION ANALYSIS ASSAY 100
pH, BLOOD

Normal values:
Arterial: 7.35-7.45
Venous: 7.32-7.42
For abnormal values, refer to ARTERIAL BLOOD GASES.

pH, URINE; SEE URINE pH
PHENOBARBITAL
Normal therapeutic range: 15-30 μg/ml for epilepsy control

PHENYTOIN (DILANTIN)
Normal therapeutic range: 10-20 μg/ml

PHOSPHATASE, ACID; SEE ACID PHOSPHATASE
PHOSPHATASE, ALKALINE; SEE ALKALINE PHOSPHATASE
PHOSPHATE (SERUM)
Normal range: 2.5-5 mg/dl
Elevated in:
a. Excessive phosphate administration
   1. Excessive oral intake or IV administration
   2. Laxatives containing phosphate (phosphate tablets, phosphate enemas)
b. Decreased renal phosphate excretion
   1. Acute or chronic renal failure
   2. Hypoparathyroidism or pseudohypoparathyroidism
   3. Acromegaly, thyrotoxicosis
   4. Biphosphonate therapy
   5. Tumor calcinosis
   6. Sickle cell anemia
c. Transcellular shift out of cells
   1. Chemotherapy of lymphoma or leukemia, tumor lysis syndrome, hemolysis.
   2. Acidosis.
   3. Rhabdomyolysis, malignant hyperthermia.
d. Artifact: in vitro hemolysis.
e. Pseudohyperphosphatemia: hyperlipidemia, paraproteinemia, hyperbilirubinemia.
Decreased in:
a. Decreased intake (prolonged starvation alcoholics], hyperalimentation, or IV infusion without phosphate
b. Malabsorption
c. Phosphate-binding antacids
d. Renal loss
   1. RTA
   2. Fanconi's syndrome, vitamin D–resistant rickets

    3. ATN (diuretic phase)
    4. Hyperparathyroidism (primary or secondary)
    5. Familial hypophosphatemia
    6. Hypokalemia, hypomagnesemia
    7. Acute volume expansion
    8. Glycosuria, idiopathic hypercalciuria
    9. Acetazolamide
 e. Transcellular shift into cells
    1. Alcohol withdrawal
    2. DKA (recovery phase)
    3. Glucose-insulin or catecholamine infusion
    4. Anabolic steroids
    5. Total parenteral nutrition
    6. Theophylline overdose
    7. Severe hyperthermia; recovery from hypothermia
    8. "Hungry bones" syndrome

PLASMINOGEN

Normal: Immunoassay (antigen): <20mg/dl
Elevated in: infection, trauma, neoplasm, myocardial infarction (acute phase reactant), pregnancy, bilirubinemia
Decreased in: DIC, severe liver disease, thrombolytic therapy with streptokinase or urokinase, alteplase therapy

PLATELET AGGREGATION

Normal: full aggregation (generally >60%) in response to epinephrine, thrombin, ristocetin, adenosine diphosphate (ADP), collagen
Elevated in: heparin therapy, hemolysis, lipemia, nicotine use, hereditary and acquired disorders of platelet adhesion, activation, and aggregation
Decreased in: drug therapy (aspirin, some penicillins, chloroquine, chlorpromazine, clofibrate, captopril), Glanzmann's thrombasthenia, Bernard-Soulier syndrome, Wiskott-Aldrich syndrome, cyclooxygenase deficiency. In von Willebrand's disease there is normal aggregation with ADP, collagen, and epinephrine use but abnormal agglutination with ristocetin use.

PLATELET ANTIBODIES

Normal: absent
Present in: ITP (>90% of patients with chronic ITP). Patients with nonimmune thrombocytopenias may have false-positive results.

PLATELET COUNT

Normal range: 130-400 $\times$ $10^3/mm^3$
Elevated in: iron deficiency, posthemorrhage, neoplasms (GI tract), chronic myelogenous leukemia (CML), polycythemia vera, myelofibrosis with myeloid metaplasia, infections, postsplenectomy, postpartum, hemophilia, pancreatitis, cirrhosis
Decreased in:
a. Increased destruction
   1. Immunologic
   2. Drug therapy: quinine, quinidine, digitalis, procainamide, thiazide diuretics, sulfonamides, phenytoin, aspirin, penicillin, heparin, gold, meprobamate, sulfa drugs, phenylbutazone, NSAIDs, methyldopa, cimetidine, furosemide, INH, cephalosporins, chlorpropamide, organic arsenicals, chloroquine, platelet glycoprotein IIb/IIIa receptor inhibitors, ranitidine, indomethacin, carboplatin, ticlopidine, clopidogrel

3. ITP
4. Transfusion reaction: transfusion of platelets with plasminogen activator (PLA) in recipients without PLA-1
5. Fetal/maternal incompatibility
6. Collagen-vascular diseases (e.g., SLE)
7. Autoimmune hemolytic anemia
8. Lymphoreticular disorders (e.g., CLL)
9. Nonimmunologic
10. Prosthetic heart valves
11. Thrombotic thrombocytopenic purpura (TTP)
12. Sepsis
13. DIC
14. Hemolytic-uremic syndrome (HUS)
15. Giant cavernous hemangioma
  b. Decreased production
1. Abnormal marrow
2. Marrow infiltration (e.g., leukemia, lymphoma, fibrosis)
3. Marrow suppression (e.g., chemotherapy, alcohol, radiation)
4. Hereditary disorders
5. Wiskott-Aldrich syndrome: X-linked disorder characterized by thrombocytopenia, eczema, and repeated infections
6. May-Hegglin anomaly: increased megakaryocytes but ineffective thrombopoiesis
7. Vitamin deficiencies (e.g., vitamin B_{12}, folic acid)
  c. Splenic sequestration, hypersplenism
  d. Dilutional, as a result of massive transfusion

PLATELET FUNCTION ANALYSIS 100 ASSAY (PFA)

Normal: This test is a two-component assay where blood is aspirated through two capillary tubes, one of which is coated with collagen and ADP (COL/ADP) and the other with collagen and epinephrine (COL/EPI). The test measures the ability of platelets to occlude an aperture in a biologically active membrane treated with COL/ADP and COL/EPI. During the test the platelets adhere to the surface of the tube and cause blood flow to cease. The closing time refers to the cessation of blood flow and is reported in conjunction with the hematocrit and platelet count. Hematocrit count must be more than 25% and platelet count less than 50,000/µl for the test to be performed.
COL/ADP: 70-120 sec
COL/EP: 75-120 sec
Elevated in: acquired platelet dysfunction, von Willebrand's disease, anemia, thrombocytopenia, use of aspirin and NSAIDs

POTASSIUM (SERUM)

Normal range: 3.5-5 mEq/L
Elevated in:
a. Pseudohyperkalemia
1. Hemolyzed specimen
2. Severe thrombocytosis (platelet count > 10^6 ml)
3. Severe leukocytosis (WBC count > 10^5 ml)
4. Fist clenching during phlebotomy
b. Excessive potassium intake (often in setting of impaired excretion)
1. Potassium replacement therapy
2. High-potassium diet
3. Salt substitutes with potassium
4. Potassium salts of antibiotics

   c. Decreased renal excretion
     1. Potassium-sparing diuretics (e.g., spironolactone, triamterene, amiloride)
     2. Renal insufficiency
     3. Mineralocorticoid deficiency
     4. Hyporeninemic hypoaldosteronism (DM)
     5. Tubular unresponsiveness to aldosterone (e.g., SLE, multiple myeloma, sickle cell disease)
     6. Type 4 RTA
     7. ACE inhibitors
     8. Heparin administration
     9. NSAIDs
     10. Trimethoprim-sulfamethoxazole
     11. Beta blockers
     12. Pentamidine
  d. Redistribution (excessive cellular release)
     1. Acidemia (each 0.1 decrease in pH increases the serum potassium by 0.4 to 0.6 mEq/L). Lactic acidosis and ketoacidosis cause minimal redistribution.
     2. Insulin deficiency
     3. Drug therapy (e.g., succinylcholine, markedly increased digitalis level, arginine, ß-adrenergic blockers)
     4. Hypertonicity
     5. Hemolysis
     6. Tissue necrosis, rhabdomyolysis, burns
     7. Hyperkalemic periodic paralysis

Decreased in:
  a. Cellular shift (redistribution) and undetermined mechanisms
     1. Alkalosis (each 0.1 increase in pH decreases serum potassium by 0.4 to 0.6 mEq/L)
     2. Insulin administration
     3. Vitamin B_{12} therapy for megaloblastic anemias, acute leukemias
     4. Hypokalemic periodic paralysis: rare familial disorder manifested by recurrent attacks of flaccid paralysis and hypokalemia.
     5. ß-Adrenergic agonists (e.g., terbutaline), decongestants, bronchodilators, theophylline, caffeine
     6. Barium poisoning, toluene intoxication, verapamil intoxication, chloroquine intoxication
     7. Correction of digoxin intoxication with digoxin antibody fragments (Digibind)
  b. Increased renal excretion
     1. Drugs
       a. Diuretics, including carbonic anhydrase inhibitors (e.g., acetazolamide)
       b. Amphotericin B
       c. High-dose sodium penicillin, nafcillin, ampicillin, or carbenicillin
       d. Cisplatin
       e. Aminoglycosides
       f. Corticosteroids, mineralocorticoids
       g. Foscarnet sodium
     2. RTA: distal (type 1) or proximal (type 2)
     3. Diabetic ketoacidosis (DKA), ureteroenterostomy
     4. Magnesium deficiency
     5. Postobstruction diuresis, diuretic phase of ATN
     6. Osmotic diuresis (e.g., mannitol)
     7. Bartter's syndrome: hyperplasia of juxtaglomerular cells leading to increased renin and aldosterone, metabolic alkalosis, hypokalemia, muscle weakness, and tetany (seen in young adults)

8. Increased mineralocorticoid activity (primary or secondary aldosteronism), Cushing's syndrome
9. Chronic metabolic alkalosis from loss of gastric fluid (increased renal potassium secretion)

c. GI loss
   1. Vomiting, nasogastric suction
   2. Diarrhea
   3. Laxative abuse
   4. Villous adenoma
   5. Fistulas

d. Inadequate dietary intake (e.g., anorexia nervosa)

e. Cutaneous loss (excessive sweating)

f. High dietary sodium intake, excessive use of licorice

POTASSIUM, URINE; SEE URINE POTASSIUM

PROCAINAMIDE

Normal therapeutic range: 4-10 μg/ml

PROGESTERONE, SERUM

Normal:

Male: 15-70 ng/dl

Female follicular phase: 15-70 ng/dl

Female luteal phase: 200-2500 ng/dl

Elevated in: congenital adrenal hyperplasia, drug therapy (clomiphene, corticosterone, 11-deoxycortisol, dihydroprogesterone), molar pregnancy, lipoid ovarian tumor

Decreased in: primary or secondary hypogonadism, oral contraceptive use, ampicillin therapy, threatened abortion

PROLACTIN

Normal range: <20 ng/ml

Elevated in: prolactinomas (level >200 highly suggestive), drug therapy (phenothiazines, cimetidine, tricyclic antidepressants, metoclopramide, estrogens, antihypertensives [methyldopa, verapamil], haloperidol), postpartum, stress, hypoglycemia, hypothyroidism

PROSTATIC SPECIFIC ANTIGEN (PSA)

Normal range: 0-4 ng/ml. It is important to remember that there is no PSA level below which prostate cancer can be ruled out, and no level above which prostate cancer is certain. The individual's PSA is only part of the equation. Other risk factors need to be considered, such as age, race, family history, findings on digital rectal examination, percent free PSA ratio, and PSA velocity (rate of change from prior PSA measurement).

Elevated in: benign prostatic hypertrophy, carcinoma of prostate, postrectal examination, prostate trauma, androgen therapy, prostatitis, urethral instrumentation.

Note: Measurement of free PSA is useful to assess the probability of prostate cancer in patients with normal digital rectal examination and total PSA between 4 and 10 ng/ml. In these patients the global risk of prostate cancer is 25% to 40%; however, if the free PSA is greater than 25%, the risk of prostate cancer decreases to 8%, whereas if the free PSA is less than 10%, the risk of cancer increases to 56%. Free PSA is also useful to evaluate the aggressiveness of prostate cancer. A low free PSA percentage generally indicates a high-grade cancer, whereas a high free PSA percentage is generally associated with a slower growing tumor.

Elevated in: drug therapy (finasteride, dutasteride, antiandrogens) bedrest

PROSTATIC ACID PHOSPHATASE
Normal: 0-0.8 U/L
Elevated in: prostate cancer (especially in metastatic prostate cancer), benign prostatic hyperplasia (BPH), prostatitis, post-prostate surgery or manipulation, hemolysis, androgen use, clofibrate therapy
Decreased in: ketoconazole use

PROTEIN (SERUM)
Normal range: 6-8 g/dl
Elevated in: dehydration, sarcoidosis, collagen-vascular diseases, multiple myeloma, Waldenström's macroglobulinemia
Decreased in: malnutrition, cirrhosis, nephrosis, low-protein diet, overhydration, malabsorption, pregnancy, severe burns, neoplasms, chronic diseases

PROTEIN C ASSAY
Normal: 70-140%
Elevated in: oral contraceptive use, stanozol therapy
Decreased in: congenital protein C deficiency, warfarin therapy, vitamin K deficiency, renal insufficiency, consumptive coagulopathies

PROTEIN ELECTROPHORESIS (SERUM)
Figure 2-12 illustrates clinicopathologic correlations with serum protein electrophoresis.

Normal range:
Albumin: 60% to 75%
Alpha$_1$: 1.7% to 5%
Alpha$_2$: 6.7% to 12.5%
Beta: 8.3% to 16.3%
Gamma: 10.7% to 20%
Albumin: 3.6-5.2 g/dl
Alpha-1: 0.1-0.4 g/dl
Alpha-2: 0.4-1.0 g/dl
Beta: 0.5-1.2 g/dl
Gamma: 0.6-1.6 g/dl
Elevated in: Albumin: dehydration
Alpha$_1$: neoplastic diseases, inflammation
Alpha$_2$: neoplasms, inflammation, infection, nephrotic syndrome
Beta: hypothyroidism, biliary cirrhosis, diabetes mellitus
Gamma: see IMMUNOGLOBULINS
Decreased in: Albumin: malnutrition, chronic liver disease, malabsorption, nephrotic syndrome, burns, SLE
Alpha$_1$: emphysema (alpha$_1$-antitrypsin deficiency), nephrosis
Alpha$_2$: hemolytic anemias (decreased haptoglobin), severe hepatocellular damage
Beta: hypocholesterolemia, nephrosis
Gamma: see IMMUNOGLOBULINS

PROTEIN S ASSAY
Normal: 65% to 140%
Elevated in: presence of lupus anticoagulant
Decreased in: hereditary deficiency, acute thrombotic events, DIC, surgery, oral contraceptive use, pregnancy, hormone replacement therapy, L-asparaginase treatment

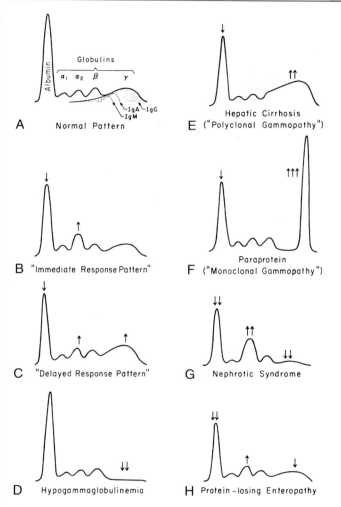

Figure 2-12 Serum protein electrophoresis: Clinicopathologic correlations. *(From Henry JB, ed: Clinical Diagnosis and Management by Laboratory Methods. Philadelphia, WB Saunders, 2001.)*

PROTHROMBIN TIME (PT)

Normal range: 11-13.2 seconds

Note: The prothrombin time is reported as absolute clotting time in seconds and also as a derivative number called International Normalized Ratio (INR). This ratio is derived from the actual PT of the patient divided by the mean PT of a group of healthy subjects. INR should always be used when interpreting prothrombin time.

Elevated in: liver disease, factor deficiency (I, II, V, VII, X), DIC, vitamin K deficiency, afibrinogenemia, dysfibrinogenemia, drug therapy (oral anticoagulant [warfarin], heparin, salicylate, chloral hydrate, diphenylhydantoin, estrogens, antacids, phenylbutazone, quinidine, antibiotics, allopurinol, anabolic steroids)

Decreased in: vitamin K supplementation, thrombophlebitis, drug therapy (gluthetimide, estrogens, griseofulvin, diphenhydramine)

PROTOPORPHYRIN (FREE ERYTHROCYTE)

Normal range: 16-36 μg/dl of RBC

Elevated in: iron deficiency, lead poisoning, sideroblastic anemias, anemia of chronic disease, hemolytic anemias, erythropoietic protoporphyria

PSA; SEE PROSTATIC-SPECIFIC ANTIGEN
PT; SEE PROTHROMBIN TIME
PTT; SEE PARTIAL THROMBOPLASTIN TIME
RDW; SEE RED BLOOD CELL DISTRIBUTION WIDTH
RED BLOOD CELL COUNT

Normal range:

Male: $4.3\text{-}5.9 \times 10^6/mm^3$

Female: $3.5\text{-}5.0 \times 10^6/mm^3$

Elevated in: hemoconcentration/dehydration, stress, polycythemia vera, smokers, high altitude, cardiovascular disease, renal cell carcinoma and other erythropoietin-producing neoplasms

Decreased in: anemias, hemolysis, chronic renal failure, hemorrhage, failure of marrow production

RED BLOOD CELL DISTRIBUTION WIDTH (RDW)

Test description: This test measures the variability of red blood cell size (anisocytosis).

Normal range: 11.5-14.5

Normal RDW and: Elevated MCV: aplastic anemia, preleukemia

Normal MCV: normal, anemia of chronic disease, acute blood loss or hemolysis, CLL, CML, nonanemic enzymopathy or hemoglobinopathy

Decreased MCV: anemia of chronic disease, heterozygous thalassemia

Elevated RDW and: Elevated MCV: vitamin B_{12} deficiency, folate deficiency, immune hemolytic anemia, cold agglutinins, CLL with high count, liver disease

Normal MCV: early iron deficiency, early vitamin B_{12} deficiency, early folate deficiency, anemic globinopathy

Decreased MCV: iron deficiency, RBC fragmentation, hemoglobin H (HbH) disease, thalassemia intermedia

RED BLOOD CELL FOLATE; SEE FOLATE, RBC
RED BLOOD CELL MASS (VOLUME)

Normal range:

Male: 20-36 ml/kg of body weight (1.15-1.21 L/m^2 body surface area [BSA])

Female: 19-31 ml/kg of body weight (0.95-1.00 L/m^2 BSA)

Elevated in: polycythemia vera, hypoxia (smokers, high altitude, cardiovascular disease), hemoglobinopathies with high oxygen affinity, erythropoietin-producing tumors (renal cell carcinoma)

Decreased in: hemorrhage, chronic disease, failure of marrow production, anemias, hemolysis

RENIN (SERUM)

Elevated in: renal hypertension, reduced plasma volume, secondary aldosteronism, drug therapy (thiazides, estrogen, minoxidil), chronic renal failure, Bartter's syndrome, pregnancy (normal), pheochromocytoma

Decreased in: primary aldosteronism, adrenocortical hypertension, increased plasma volume, drug therapy (propranolol, reserpine, clonidine)

RESPIRATORY SYNCYTIAL VIRUS (RSV) SCREEN

Test description: PCR test can be performed on nasopharyngeal swab, wash, or aspirate

RETICULOCYTE COUNT

Normal range: 0.5% to 1.5%

Elevated in: hemolytic anemia (sickle cell crisis, thalassemia major, autoimmune hemolysis), hemorrhage, postanemia therapy (folic acid, ferrous sulfate, vitamin B_{12}), chronic renal failure

Decreased in: aplastic anemia, marrow suppression (sepsis, chemotherapeutic agents, radiation), hepatic cirrhosis, blood transfusion, anemias of disordered maturation (iron deficiency anemia, megaloblastic anemia, sideroblastic anemia, anemia of chronic disease)

RHEUMATOID FACTOR

Normal: negative

Present in titer. 1:20: rheumatoid arthritis, SLE, chronic inflammatory processes, old age, infections, liver disease, multiple myeloma, sarcoidosis, pulmonary fibrosis, Sjögren's syndrome

Table 2-5 describes the sensitivity and specificity of rheumatoid factor.

RNP; SEE EXTRACTABLE NUCLEAR ANTIGEN
ROTAVIRUS SEROLOGY

Test description: PCR test is performed on a stool specimen.

SCHILLING TEST; SEE Figure 2-13.

SEDIMENTATION RATE; SEE ERYTHROCYTE SEDIMENTATION RATE
SEMEN ANALYSIS

Normal: Volume: 2-6 ml
Sperm density: >20 million/ml
Total number of spermatozoa: >80 million/ejaculate
Progressive motility score evaluated 2 to 4 hours after ejaculate: 3-4
Live spermatozoa: ≥50% of total
Normal spermatozoa: ≥0% of total
Immature forms: <4%

Decreased in: cryptorchidism, testicular failure, obstruction of ejaculatory system, postvasectomy, drug therapy (cimetidine, ketoconazole, nitrofurantion, cancer chemotherapy agents, sulfasalazine), testicular radiation

TABLE 2-5 Sensitivity and Specificity of Rheumatoid Factor

Diagnosis	≥150 U/ml	≥50 U/ml	≥100 U/ml
Rheumatoid arthritis	66*	46	26
Sjögren's syndrome	62	52	33
Systemic lupus erythematosus	27	10	3
Mixed connective tissue disease	23	13	6
Scleroderma	44	18	2
Polymyositis	18	0	0
Reactive arthritis	0	0	0
Osteoarthritis	25	4	4
Healthy controls	13	0	0
Sensitivity (%)	66	46	26
Specificity (%)	74	88 (92†)	95 (98†)

*Percentage of positive patients.
† Specificity when a diagnosis of Sjögren's syndrome can be excluded.
Rheumatoid factors were determined by nephelometry in 100 patients with RA, in more than 200 patients with other rheumatic diseases, and in 30 healthy control persons.
From Hochberg MC, et al, eds: *Rheumatology*, ed 3, St. Louis, Mosby, 2003.

SGOT; SEE ASPARTATE AMINOTRANSFERASE
SGPT; SEE ALANINE AMINOTRANSFERASE
SICKLE CELL TEST
Normal: negative
Positive in: sickle cell anemia, sickle cell trait, combination of Hb S gene with other disorders such as alpha thalassemia, beta thalassemia

SMOOTH MUSCLE ANTIBODY
Normal: negative
Present in: chronic active hepatitis (≥1:80), primary biliary cirrhosis (≥1:80), infectious mononucleosis

SODIUM (SERUM)
Normal range: 135-147 mEq/L
Elevated in:
a. Isovolemic hypernatremia (decreased total body water [TBW], normal total body sodium [TBNa], and extra cellular fluid [ECF])
   1. DI (neurogenic and nephrogenic)
   2. Skin loss (hyperhemia), iatrogenic, reset osmostat
b. Hypervolemic hypernatremia (increased TBW, markedly increased TBNa and ECF)
   1. Iatrogenic (administration of hypernatremic solutions)
   2. Mineralocorticoid excess (Conn's syndrome, Cushing's syndrome)
   3. Salt ingestion
c. Hypovolemic hypernatremia (loss of H_2O and Na^+ (H_2O loss > Na^+))
   1. Renal losses (e.g., diuretics, glycosuria)
   2. GI, respiratory, skin losses
   3. Adrenal deficiencies

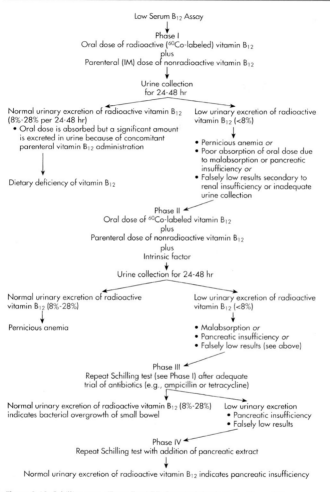

Figure 2-13 Schilling test. *(From Ferri FF: Practical Guide to the Care of the Medical Patient, ed 7, St. Louis, Mosby, 2007.)*

Decreased in:
a. Hypotonic hyponatremia
b. Isovolemic hyponatremia
   1. SIADH
   2. Water intoxication (e.g., schizophrenia, primary polydipsia, sodium-free irrigant solutions, multiple tap-water enemas, dilute infant formulas). These

entities are rare and often associated with a deranged ADH axis.
3. Renal failure
4. Reset osmostat (e.g., chronic active TB, carcinomatosis)
5. Glucocorticoid deficiency (hypopituitarism)
6. Hypothyroidism
7. Thiazide diuretics, NSAIDs, carbamazepine, amitriptyline, thioridazine, vincristine, cyclophosphamide, colchicine, tolbutamide, chlorpropamide, ACE inhibitors, clofibrate, oxytocin, selective serotonin reuptake inhibitors (SSRIs), amiodarone. With these medications, various drug-induced mechanisms are involved.
c. Hypovolemic hyponatremia
1. Renal losses (diuretics, partial urinary tract obstruction, salt-losing renal disease)
2. Extrarenal losses: GI (vomiting, diarrhea), extensive burns, third spacing (peritonitis, pancreatitis)
3. Adrenal insufficiency
d. Hypervolemic hyponatremia
1. CHF
2. Nephrotic syndrome
3. Cirrhosis
4. Pregnancy
e. **Isotonic hyponatremia** (normal serum osmolality)
1. Pseudohyponatremia (increased serum lipids and serum proteins). Newer sodium assays eliminate this problem.
2. Isotonic infusion (e.g., glucose, mannitol)
f. **Hypertonic hyponatremia** (increased serum osmolality)
1. Hyperglycemia: Each 100 ml/dl increment in blood sugar above normal decreases plasma sodium concentration by 1.6 mEq/L.
2. Hypertonic infusions (e.g., glucose, mannitol)

STREPTOZYME; SEE ANTISTREPTOLYSIN O TITER

SUCROSE HEMOLYSIS TEST (SUGAR WATER TEST)
Normal: absence of hemolysis
Positive in: paroxysmal nocturnal hemoglobinuria (PNH)
False positive: autoimmune hemolytic anemia, megaloblastic anemias
False negative: may occur with use of heparin or EDTA

SUDAN III STAIN (QUALITATIVE SCREENING FOR FECAL FAT)
Normal: negative. This test should be preceded by diet containing 100 to 150 g of dietary fat per day for 1 week, avoidance of a high-fiber diet, and avoidance of suppositories or oily material before specimen collection.
Positive in: steatorrhea, use of castor oil or mineral oil droplets

T_3 (TRIIODOTHYRONINE)
Normal range: 75-220 ng/dl
Abnormal values:
a. Elevated in hyperthyroidism (usually earlier and to a greater extent than serum T_4).
b. Useful in diagnosing:
1. T_3 hyperthyroidism (thyrotoxicosis): increased T_3, normal FTI
2. Toxic nodular goiter: increased T_3, normal or increased T_4
3. Iodine deficiency: normal T_3, possibly decreased T_4
4. Thyroid replacement therapy with liothyronine (Cytomel): normal T_4, increased T_3 if patient is symptomatically hyperthyroid

c. Not ordered routinely but indicated when hyperthyroidism is suspected and serum free T_4 or FTI inconclusive.

T_3 RESIN UPTAKE (T_3RU)
Normal range: 25% to 35%
Abnormal values: Increased in hyperthyroidism. T_3 resin uptake (T_3RU or RT$_3$U) measures the percentage of free T_4 (not bound to protein); it does not measure serum T_3 concentration; T_3RU and other tests that reflect thyroid hormone binding to plasma protein are also known as thyroid hormone-binding ratios (THBR).

T_4, Serum T_4, and FREE (FREE THYROXINE)
Normal range: 0.8-2.8 ng/dl
Abnormal values: serum thyroxine (T_4)
Elevated in:
1. Graves' disease
2. Toxic multinodular goiter
3. Toxic adenoma
4. Iatrogenic and factitious
5. Transient hyperthyroidism
   a. Subacute thyroiditis
   b. Hashimoto's thyroiditis
   c. Silent thyroiditis
6. Rare causes: hypersecretion of TSH (e.g., pituitary neoplasms), struma ovarii, ingestion of large amounts of iodine in a patient with preexisting thyroid hyperplasia or adenoma (Jod-Basedow phenomenon), hydatidiform mole, carcinoma of thyroid, amiodarone therapy of arrhythmias

Serum thyroxine test measures both circulating thyroxine bound to protein (represents > 99% of circulating T_4) and unbound (free) thyroxine. Values vary with protein binding; changes in the concentration of T_4 secondary to changes in thyroxine-binding globulin (TBG) can be caused by the following:

Increased TBG ($\uparrow T_4$)	Decreased TBG ($\downarrow T_4$)
Pregnancy	Androgens, glucocorticoids
Estrogens	Nephrotic syndrome, cirrhosis
Acute infectious hepatitis	Acromegaly
Oral contraceptives	Hypoproteinemia
Familial	Familial
Fluorouracil, clofibrate, heroin, methadone	Phenytoin, acetylsalicylic acid (ASA) and other NSAIDs, high-dose penicillin, asparaginase
Chronic debilitating illness	

To eliminate the suspected influence of protein binding on thyroxine values, two additional tests are available: T_3 resin uptake and serum free thyroxine.

Serum free T_4
Elevated in: Graves' disease, toxic multinodular goiter, toxic adenoma, iatrogenic and factitious causes, transient hyperthyroidism
Serum free T_4 directly measures unbound thyroxine. Free T_4 can be measured by equilibrium dialysis (gold standard of free T_4 assays) or by immunometric techniques (influenced by serum levels of lipids, proteins, and certain drugs). The free thyroxine index can also be easily calculated by multiplying T_4 times T_3RU

and dividing the result by 100; the FTI corrects for any abnormal T_4 values secondary to protein binding:

$$FTI = T_4 \times T_3RU/100$$
Normal values equal 1.1 to 4.3

TEGRETOL; SEE CARBAMAZEPINE

TESTOSTERONE
Elevated in: adrenogenital syndrome, polycystic ovarian syndrome
Decreased in: Klinefelter's syndrome, male hypogonadism

THEOPHYLLINE
Normal therapeutic range: 10-20 μg/ml

THIAMINE
Normal: 275-675 ng/g
Elevated in: polycythemia vera, leukemia, Hodgkin's disease
Decreased in: alcoholism, dietary deficiency, excessive consumption of tea (contains antithiamine factor) or raw fish (contains a microbial thiaminase), chronic illness, prolonged illness, barbiturates

THORACENTESIS FLUID

Testing and evaluation of results:
1. Pleural effusion fluid should be differentiated in exudate or transudate. The initial laboratory studies should be aimed only at distinguishing an exudate from a transudate.
    a. Tube 1: protein, LDH, albumin.
    b. Tubes 2, 3, 4: Save the fluid until further notice. In selected patients with suspected empyema, a pH level may be useful (generally $\leq$ 7.0). See the following for proper procedure to obtain a pH level from pleural fluid.
    Note: Do not order further tests until the presence of an exudate is confirmed on the basis of protein and LDH determinations (see Section III, Pleural Effusion); however, if the results of protein and LDH determinations cannot be obtained within a reasonable time (resulting in unnecessary delay), additional laboratory tests should be ordered at the time of thoracentesis.
2. A serum/effusion albumin gradient of 1.2 g/dl or less is indicative of exudative effusions, especially in patients with CHF treated with diuretics.
3. Note the appearance of the fluid:
    a. A grossly hemorrhagic effusion can be a result of a traumatic tap, neoplasm, or an embolus with infarction.
    b. A milky appearance indicates either of the following:
        1. Chylous effusion: caused by trauma or tumor invasion of the thoracic duct; lipoprotein electrophoresis of the effusion reveals chylomicrons and triglyceride levels greater than 115 mg/dl.
        2. Pseudochylous effusion: often seen with chronic inflammation of the pleural space (e.g., TB, connective tissue diseases).
4. If transudate, consider CHF, cirrhosis, chronic renal failure, and other hypoproteinemic states and perform subsequent workup accordingly.
5. If exudate, consider ordering these tests on the pleural fluid:
    a. Cytologic examination for malignant cells (for suspected neoplasm)
    b. Gram stain, cultures (aerobic and anaerobic), and sensitivities (for suspected infectious process)
    c. AFB stain and cultures (for suspected TB)

d. pH: a value less than 7.0 suggests parapneumonic effusion or empyema; a pleural fluid pH must be drawn anaerobically and iced immediately; the syringe should be prerinsed with 0.2 ml of 1:1000 heparin.
e. Glucose: a low glucose level suggests parapneumonic effusions and rheumatoid arthritis.
f. Amylase: a high amylase level suggests pancreatitis or ruptured esophagus.
g. Perplexing pleural effusions are often a result of malignancy (e.g., lymphoma, malignant mesothelioma, ovarian carcinoma), TB, subdiaphragmatic processes, prior asbestos exposure, or postcardiac injury syndrome.

THROMBIN TIME (TT)
Normal range: 11.3-18.5 seconds
Elevated in: thrombolytic and heparin therapy, DIC, hypofibrinogenemia, dysfibrinogenemia

THYROGLOBULIN
Normal: 3-40 ng/ml. Thyroglobulin is a tumor marker for monitoring the status of patients with papillary or follicular thyroid cancer following resection.
Elevated in: papillary or follicular thyroid cancer, Hashimoto's thyroiditis, Graves' disease, subacute thyroiditis

THYROID MICROSOMAL ANTIBODIES
Normal: Undetectable. Low titers may be present in 5% to 10% of normal individuals.
Elevated in: Hashimoto's disease, thyroid carcinoma, early hypothyroidism, pernicious anemia

THYROID-STIMULATING HORMONE (TSH)
Normal range: 2-11.0 μU/ml
Elevated in:
1. Primary hypothyroidism (thyroid gland dysfunction): cause of more than 90% of cases of hypothyroidism
   a. Hashimoto's thyroiditis (chronic lymphocytic thyroiditis); most common cause of hypothyroidism after 8 years of age
   b. Idiopathic myxedema (possibly a nongoitrous form of Hashimoto's thyroiditis)
   c. Previous treatment of hyperthyroidism (^{131}I therapy, subtotal thyroidectomy)
   d. Subacute thyroiditis
   e. Radiation therapy of the neck (usually for malignant disease)
   f. Iodine deficiency or excess
   g. Drug therapy (lithium, PAS, sulfonamides, phenylbutazone, amiodarone, thiourea)
   h. Congenital (approximately 1:4000 live births)
   i. Prolonged treatment with iodides
2. Tissue resistance to thyroid hormone (rare)
   TSH is used primarily to diagnose hypothyroidism (the increased TSH level is the earliest thyroid abnormality detected); conventional TSH radioimmunoassays have been replaced by new third-generation TSH radioimmunoassays, which are useful to detect both clinical or subclinical thyroid hormone excess or deficiency. Various factors can influence TSH levels (recovery from severe illness and metoclopramide, chlorpromazine, haloperidol, and amiodarone use all elevate TSH; dopamine and corticosteroid therapies lower it). Apparently healthy ambulatory patients with

subnormal TSH levels should be checked with measurement of free T_4 and total T_3. If they are normal, a T_3 level (by trace equilibrium dialysis) should be obtained to distinguish subclinical hyperthyroidism from overt free T_3 toxicosis.

Decreased in: hyperthyroidism, secondary hypothyroidism (pituitary dysfunction, postpartum necrosis, neoplasm, infiltrative disease causing deficiency of TSH), tertiary hypothyroidism (hypothalamic disease [granuloma, neoplasm, or irradiation causing deficiency of TSH])

THYROTROPIN (TSH) RECEPTOR ANTIBODIES

Normal: <130% of basal activity

Elevated in: Values between 1.3 and 2.0 are found in 10% of patients with thyroid disease other than Graves' disease. Values greater than 2.8 have been found only in patients with Graves' disease.

THYROTROPIN-RELEASING HORMONE (TRH) STIMULATION TEST

Elevated in: celiac disease (specificity 94%-97%, sensitivity 90%-98%), dermatitis herpetiformis

TIBC; SEE IRON-BINDING CAPACITY

TISSUE TRANSGLUTAMINASE ANTIBODY

Normal: negative

Present in: celiac disease (specificity 94%-97%, sensitivity 90%-98%), dermatitis herpetiformis

TRANSFERRIN

Normal range: 170-370 mg/dl

Elevated in: iron deficiency anemia, oral contraceptive administration, viral hepatitis, late pregnancy

Decreased in: nephrotic syndrome, liver disease, hereditary deficiency, protein malnutrition, neoplasms, chronic inflammatory states, chronic illness, thalassemia, hemochromatosis, hemolytic anemia

TRIGLYCERIDES

Normal range: <160 mg/dl

Elevated in: hyperlipoproteinemias (types I, IIb, III, IV, V), diet high in saturated fats, hypothyroidism, pregnancy, estrogen therapy, pancreatitis, alcohol intake, nephrotic syndrome, poorly controlled diabetes mellitus, sedentary lifestyle, glycogen storage disease

Decreased in: malnutrition, vigorous exercise, congenital abetalipoproteinemias, drug therapy (gemfibrozil, fenofibrate nicotinic acid, metformin, clofibrate)

TRIIODOTHYRONINE; SEE T_3

TROPONINS, SERUM

Normal range: 0-0.4 ng/ml (negative). If there is clinical suspicion of evolving acute MI or ischemic episode, repeat testing in 5 to 6 hours is recommended.

Indeterminate: 0.05-0.49 ng/ml. Suggest further tests. In a patient with unstable angina and this troponin I level, there is an increased risk of a cardiac event in the near future.

Strong probability of acute MI: ≥ 0.50 ng/ml

Cardiac troponin T (cTnT) is a highly sensitive marker for myocardial injury for the first 48 hours after MI and for up to 5 to 7 days (see Figure 2-2). It may be also elevated in renal failure, chronic muscle disease, and trauma.

Cardiac troponin I (cTnI) is highly sensitive and specific for myocardial injury (≥ CK-MB) in the initial 8 hours, peaks within 24 hours, and lasts up to 7 days. With progressively higher levels of cTnI, the risk of mortality increases because the amount of necrosis increases.

Elevated in: In addition to acute coronary syndrome, many diseases such as sepsis, hypovolemia, atrial fibrillation, congestive heart failure, pulmonary embolism, myocarditis, myocardial contusion, and renal failure can be associated with an increase in troponin level.

TSH; SEE THYROID-STIMULATING HORMONE

TT; SEE THROMBIN TIME

UNCONJUGATED BILIRUBIN; SEE BILIRUBIN, INDIRECT

UREA NITROGEN

Normal range: 8-18 mg/dl

Elevated in: dehydration, renal disease (glomerulonephritis, pyelonephritis, diabetic nephropathy), urinary tract obstruction (prostatic hypertrophy), drug therapy (aminoglycosides and other antibiotics, diuretics, lithium, corticosteroids), gastrointestinal bleeding, decreased renal blood flow (shock, CHF, MI)

Decreased in: liver disease, malnutrition, third trimester of pregnancy

URIC ACID (SERUM)

Normal range: 2-7 mg/dl

Elevated in: hereditary enzyme deficiency (hypoxanthine-guanine-phosphoribosyl transferase), renal failure, gout, excessive cell lysis (chemotherapeutic agents, radiation therapy, leukemia, lymphoma, hemolytic anemia), acidosis, myeloproliferative disorders, diet high in purines or protein, drug therapy (diuretics, low doses of ASA, ethambutol, nicotinic acid), lead poisoning, hypothyroidism

Decreased in: drug therapy (allopurinol, high doses of ASA, probenecid, warfarin, corticosteroid), deficiency of xanthine oxidase, SIADH, renal tubular deficits (Fanconi's syndrome), alcoholism, liver disease, diet deficient in protein or purines, Wilson's disease, hemochromatosis

URINALYSIS

Normal range:

　　Color: light straw
　　Appearance: clear
　　pH: 4.5-8.0 (average, 6.0)
　　Specific gravity: 1.005-1.030
　　Protein: absent
　　Ketones: absent
　　Glucose: absent
　　Occult blood: absent

Microscopic examination:

　　RBC: 0-5 (high-power field)
　　WBC: 0-5 (high-power field)
　　Bacteria (spun specimen): absent
　　Casts: 0-4 hyaline (low-power field)

URINE AMYLASE

Normal range: 35-260 U Somogyi/hr

Elevated in: pancreatitis, carcinoma of the pancreas

URINE BILE

Normal: absent

Abnormal: Urine bilirubin: hepatitis (viral, toxic, drug-induced), biliary obstruction
Urine urobilinogen: hepatitis (viral, toxic, drug-induced), hemolytic jaundice, liver cell dysfunction (cirrhosis, infection, metastases)

URINE CALCIUM

Normal: 6.2 mmol/dl (<250 mg/24h)

Elevated in: primary hyperparathyroidism, hypervitaminosis D, bone metastases, multiple myeloma, increased calcium intake, steroids, prolonged immobilization, sarcoidosis, Paget's disease, idiopathic hypercalciuria, renal tubular acidosis

Decreased in: hypoparathyroidism, pseudohypoparathyroidism, vitamin D deficiency, vitamin D–resistant rickets, diet low in calcium, drug therapy (thiazide diuretics, oral contraceptives), familial hypocalciuric hypercalcemia, renal osteodystrophy, potassium citrate therapy

URINE cAMP

Elevated in: hypercalciuria, familial hypocalciuric hypercalcemia, primary hyperparathyroidism, pseudohypoparathyroidism, rickets

Decreased in: vitamin D intoxication, sarcoidosis

URINE CATECHOLAMINES

Normal range:

Norepinephrine: <100 μg/24 hr
Epinephrine: <10 μg/24 hr

Elevated in: pheochromocytoma, neuroblastoma, severe stress

URINE CHLORIDE

Normal range: 110-250 mEq/day

Elevated in: corticosteroids, Bartter's syndrome, diuretics, metabolic acidosis, severe hypokalemia

Decreased in: chloride depletion (vomiting), colonic villous adenoma, chronic renal failure, renal tubular acidosis

URINE COPPER

Normal range: <40 μg/24 hr

URINE CORTISOL, FREE

Normal range: 10-110 μg/24 hr

Elevated in: refer to CORTISOL (SERUM)

URINE CREATININE (24 hour)

Normal range:

Male: 0.8-1.8 g/day
Female: 0.6-1.6 g/day
Note: Useful test as an indicator of completeness of 24-hour urine collection.

URINE CRYSTALS

Uric acid: acid urine, hyperuricosuria, uric acid nephropathy
Sulfur: antibiotics containing sulfa
Calcium oxalate: ethylene glycol poisoning, acid urine, hyperoxaluria
Calcium phosphate: alkaline urine
Cystine: cystinuria

URINE EOSINOPHILS

Normal: absent
Present: interstitial nephritis, ATN, UTI, kidney transplant rejection, hepatorenal syndrome

URINE GLUCOSE (QUALITATIVE)

Normal: absent
Present in: diabetes mellitus, renal glycosuria (decreased renal threshold for glucose), glucose intolerance

URINE HEMOGLOBIN, FREE

Normal: absent
Present in: hemolysis (with saturation of serum haptoglobin binding capacity and renal threshold for tubular absorption of hemoglobin)

URINE HEMOSIDERIN

Normal: absent
Present in: PNH, chronic hemolytic anemia, hemochromatosis, blood transfusion, thalassemias

URINE 5-HYDROXYINDOLE-ACETIC ACID (URINE 5-HIAA)

Normal range: 2-8 mg/24 hr
Elevated in: carcinoid tumors, ingestion of certain foods (bananas, plums, tomatoes, avocados, pineapples, eggplant, walnuts), drug therapy (monoamine oxidase [MAO] inhibitors, phenacetin, methyldopa, glycerol guaiacolate, acetaminophen, salicylates, phenothiazines, imipramine, methocarbamol, reserpine, methamphetamine)

URINE INDICAN

Normal: absent
Present in: malabsorption resulting from intestinal bacterial overgrowth

URINE KETONES (SEMIQUANTITATIVE)

Normal: absent
Present in: DKA, alcoholic ketoacidosis, starvation, isopropanol ingestion

URINE METANEPHRINES

Normal range: 0-2.0 mg/24 hr
Elevated in: pheochromocytoma, neuroblastoma, caffeine use, drug therapy (phenothiazines, MAO inhibitors), stress

URINE MYOGLOBIN

Normal: absent
Present in: severe trauma, hyperthermia, polymyositis or dermatomyositis, carbon monoxide poisoning, drug use (narcotic and amphetamine toxicity), hypothyroidism, muscle ischemia

URINE NITRITE

Normal: absent
Present in: urinary tract infections

URINE OCCULT BLOOD

Normal: negative

Positive in: trauma to urinary tract, renal disease (glomerulonephritis, pyelonephritis), renal or ureteral calculi, bladder lesions (carcinoma, cystitis), prostatitis, prostatic carcinoma, menstrual contamination, hematopoietic disorders (hemophilia, thrombocytopenia), anticoagulant therapy, ASA use

Note: Hematuria without erythrocyte casts or significant albuminuria suggests the possibility of renal or bladder cancers.

URINE OSMOLALITY

Normal range: 50-1200 mOsm/kg

Elevated in: SIADH, dehydration, glycosuria, adrenal insufficiency, high-protein diet

Decreased in: diabetes insipidus, excessive water intake, IV hydration with D5W, acute renal insufficiency, glomerulonephritis

URINE pH

Normal range: 4.6-8.0 (average 6.0)

Elevated in: bacteriuria, vegetarian diet, renal failure with inability to form ammonia, drug therapy (antibiotics, sodium bicarbonate, acetazolamide)

Decreased in: acidosis (metabolic, respiratory), drug therapy (ammonium chloride, methenamine mandelate), diabetes mellitus, starvation, diarrhea

URINE PHOSPHATE

Normal range: 0.8-2.0 g/24 hr

Elevated in: ATN (diuretic phase), chronic renal disease, uncontrolled diabetes mellitus, hyperparathyroidism, hypomagnesemia, metabolic acidosis, metabolic alkalosis, neurofibromatosis, adult-onset vitamin D–resistant hypophosphatemic osteomalacia

Decreased in: acromegaly, acute renal failure, decreased dietary intake, hypoparathyroidism, respiratory acidosis

URINE POTASSIUM

Normal range: 25-100 mEq/24 hr

Elevated in: aldosteronism (primary, secondary), glucocorticoids therapy, alkalosis, renal tubular acidosis, excessive dietary potassium intake

Decreased in: acute renal failure, potassium-sparing diuretic use, diarrhea, hypokalemia

URINE PROTEIN (QUANTITATIVE)

Normal range: <150 mg/24 hr

Elevated in: renal disease (glomerular, tubular, interstitial), CHF, hypertension, neoplasms of renal pelvis and bladder, multiple myeloma, Waldenström's macroglobulinemia

URINE SODIUM (QUANTITATIVE)

Normal range: 40-220 mEq/day

Elevated in: diuretic administration; high sodium intake; salt-losing nephritis; acute tubular necrosis; vomiting; Addison's disease; SIADH; hypothyroidism; CHF; hepatic failure; chronic renal failure; Bartter's syndrome; glucocorticoid deficiency; interstitial nephritis caused by analgesic abuse; mannitol, dextran, or glycerol therapy; milk-alkali syndrome; decreased renin secretion; postobstructive diuresis

Decreased in: increased aldosterone, glucocorticoid excess, hyponatremia, prerenal azotemia, decreased salt intake

URINE SPECIFIC GRAVITY

Normal range: 1.005-1.03

Elevated in: dehydration, excessive fluid losses (vomiting, diarrhea, fever), ingestions of radiograph contrast media, diabetes mellitus, CHF, SIADH, adrenal insufficiency, decreased fluid intake

Decreased in: diabetes insipidus, renal disease (glomerulonephritis, pyelonephritis), excessive fluid intake or IV hydration

URINE VANILLYLMANDELIC ACID (VMA)

Normal range: <6.8 mg/24 hr

Elevated in: pheochromocytoma; neuroblastoma; ganglioblastoma; drug therapy (isoproterenol, methocarbamol, levodopa, sulfonamides, chlorpromazine); severe stress; ingestion of bananas, chocolate, vanilla, tea, coffee

Decreased in: drug therapy (MAO inhibitors, reserpine, guanethidine, methyldopa)

VARICELLA-ZOSTER VIRUS (VZV) SEROLOGY

Test description: This test can be performed on whole blood, tissue, skin lesions, and CSF.

VASOACTIVE INTESTINAL PEPTIDE (VIP)

Normal: <50 pg/ml

Elevated in: pancreatic VIPomas, neuroblastoma, pancreatic islet call hyperplasia, liver disease, multiple endocrine neoplasia (MEN) I, ganglioneuroma, ganglioneuroblastoma

VENEREAL DISEASE RESEARCH LABORATORIES (VDRL)

Normal range: negative

Positive test: syphilis, other treponemal diseases (yaws, pinta, bejel).

Note: A false-positive test may be seen in patients with SLE and other autoimmune diseases, infectious mononucleosis, HIV, atypical pneumonia, malaria, leprosy, typhus fever, rat-bite fever, or relapsing fever.

VIP; SEE VASOACTIVE INTESTINAL PEPTIDE
VISCOSITY (SERUM)

Normal range: 1.4-1.8 relative to water (1.10-1.22 centipoise)

Elevated in: monoclonal gammopathies (Waldenström's macroglobulinemia, multiple myeloma), hyperfibrinogenemia, SLE, rheumatoid arthritis, polycythemia, leukemia

VITAMIN B$_{12}$

Decreased in: pernicious anemia, dietary (strict lacto-ovo vegetarians, food faddists), malabsorption (achlorhydria, gastrectomy, ileal resection, Crohn's disease of terminal ileum, pancreatic insufficiency, drug therapy [omeprazole and other protein pump inhibitors (PPIs), metformin, cholestyramine]), chronic alcoholism, H. pylori infection

VITAMIN D, 1,25 DIHYDROXY CALCIFEROL

Normal: 16-65 pg/ml

Elevated in: tumor calcinosis, primary hyperparathyroidism, sarcoidosis, tuberculosis, idiopathic hypercalciuria

Decreased in: postmenopausal osteoporosis, chronic renal failure, hypoparathyroidism, tumor-induced osteomalacia, rickets, tumor-induced osteomalacia, elevated blood lead levels

VITAMIN K

Normal: 0.10-2.20 ng/ml
Decreased in: Primary biliary cirrhosis, anticoagulants, antibiotics, cholestyramine, GI disease, pancreatic disease, cystic fibrosis, obstructive jaundice, hypoprothrombinemia, hemorrhagic disease of the newborn

VON WILLEBRAND'S FACTOR

Normal: Levels vary according to blood type:
Blood type O: 50-150 U/dl
Blood type non-O: 90-200 U/dl
Decreased in: von Willebrand's disease (however, in type II von Willebrand's disease the antigen may be normal but the function impaired)

WBCs; SEE COMPLETE BLOOD CELL COUNT

WESTERGREN; SEE ERYTHROCYTE SEDIMENTATION RATE

WHITE BLOOD CELL COUNT; SEE COMPLETE BLOOD CELL COUNT

d-XYLOSE ABSORPTION

Normal range: 21% to 31% excreted in 5 hours
Decreased in: malabsorption syndrome

REFERENCES

1. Dhingra R et al: C-reactive protein, inflammatory conditions, and cardiovascular disease risk, *Am J Med* 120:1054-1062, 2007.
2. Jeremias A, Gibson M: Narrative review: Alternative cause for elevated cardiac troponin levels when acute coronary syndromes are excluded, *Ann Intern Med* 142:786-791, 2005.
3. Jones JS: Four no more: The PSA cutoff era is over. *Cleveland Clin J Med* 75:30-32, 2008.
4. McKie PM, Burnett JC: B-type natriuretic peptide as a marker beyond heart failure: Speculations and opportunities, *Mayo Clin Proc* 80(8):1029-1036, 2005.
5. Pagana KD, Pagana, TJ: *Mosby's Diagnostic and Laboratory Test Reference,* ed 8, St. Louis, Mosby, 2007.
6. Sarmak MJ et al: Cystatin C concentration as a risk factor for heart failure in older adults, *Ann Intern Med* 142:497-505, 2005.
7. Wu AHB: *Tietz Clinical Guide to Laboratory Tests,* Philadelphia, WB Saunders, 2006.

Diseases and Disorders

This section includes the diagnostic modalities (imaging and laboratory tests) and algorithms useful to diagnose the following 231 diseases and disorders. It is assumed that the patient has had a detailed history and physical examination before any testing sequence is initiated.

These algorithms are designed to assist clinicians in the evaluation and treatment of patients. They may not apply to all patients with a particular disease or disorder, and they are not intended to replace a clinician's individual judgment. Please note that specific findings in the patient's history and physical examination may significantly alter any of the proposed testing sequences.

44. Carcinoid syndrome   p.
45. Cardiomegaly on chest radiograph   p.
46. Cat-scratch disease   p.
47. Cavernous sinus thrombosis   p.
48. Celiac disease   p.
49. Cerebrovascular accident (CVA) (stroke)   p.
50. Cholangitis   p.
51. Cholecystitis   p.
52. Cholelithiasis   p.
53. Claudication   p.
54. Constipation   p.
55. CPK elevation   p.
56. Cushing's syndrome   p.
57. Cyanosis   p.
58. Deep vein thrombosis (DVT)   p.
59. Delirium   p.
60. Diabetes insipidus   p.
61. Diarrhea   p.
62. Disseminated intravascular coagulation (DIC)   p.
63. Diverticulitis   p.
64. Dyspepsia   p.
65. Dysphagia   p.
66. Dyspnea   p.
67. Dysuria   p.
68. Echinococcosis   p.
69. Ectopic pregnancy   p.
70. Edema, generalized   p.
71. Edema, lower extremity   p.
72. Endocarditis, infective   p.
73. Endometriosis   p.
74. Enuresis   p.
75. Epiglottitis   p.
76. Esophageal perforation   p.
77. Fatigue   p.
78. Fever of undetermined origin (FUO)   p.
79. Genital lesions/ulcers   p.
80. Goiter   p.
81. Gout   p.
82. Gynecomastia   p.
83. Hearing loss   p.
84. Hematuria   p.
85. Hemochromatosis   p.
86. Hemophilia   p.
87. Hemoptysis   p.
88. Hepatitis A   p.
89. Hepatitis B, acute   p.
90. Hepatitis C   p.
91. Hepatomegaly   p.
92. Hepatorenal syndrome   p.
93. Hirsutism   p.
94. Hydrocephalus, normal pressure (NPH)   p.
95. Hypercalcemia   p.
96. Hyperkalemia   p.
97. Hypermagnesemia   p.
98. Hypernatremia   p.
99. Hyperphosphatemia   p.

156. Peripheral arterial disease   p.
157. Peripheral nerve dysfunction   p.
158. Perirectal abscess   p.
159. Pheochromocytoma   p.
160. Pituitary adenoma   p.
161. Placenta previa   p.
162. Pleural effusion   p.
163. Polyarteritis nodosa   p.
164. Polycystic kidney disease   p.
165. Polycythemia vera   p.
166. Portal hypertension   p.
167. Portal vein thrombosis   p.
168. Prolactinoma   p.
169. Prostate cancer   p.
170. Proteinuria   p.
171. Pruritus, generalized   p.
172. Pseudomembranous colitis   p.
173. Puberty, delayed   p.
174. Puberty, precocious   p.
175. Pulmonary embolism   p.
176. Pulmonary hypertension   p.
177. Pulmonary nodule   p.
178. Purpura   p.
179. Reflex sympathetic dystrophy (RSD)   p.
180. Renal artery stenosis   p.
181. Renal insufficiency   p.
182. Renal mass   p.
183. Renal vein thrombosis   p.
184. Respiratory acidosis   p.
185. Respiratory alkalosis   p.
186. Retropharyngeal abscess   p.
187. Rhabdomyolysis   p.
188. Rotator cuff tear   p.
189. Sacroiliac joint pain   p.
190. Salivary gland neoplasm   p.
191. Sarcoidosis   p.
192. Scrotal mass   p.
193. Seizure disorder   p.
194. SIADH (syndrome of inappropriate antidiuretic hormone secretion)   p.
195. Sialolithiasis   p.
196. Sinusitis   p.
197. Small-bowel obstruction   p.
198. Spinal epidural abscess   p.
199. Spinal stenosis   p.
200. Splenomegaly   p.
201. Subarachnoid hemorrhage   p.
202. Subclavian steal syndrome   p.
203. Subdural hematoma   p.
204. Superior vena cava syndrome   p.
205. Syncope   p.
206. Temporal arteritis   p.
207. Temporomandibular joint (TMJ) syndrome   p.
208. Testicular neoplasm   p.
209. Testicular torsion   p.
210. Thoracic outlet syndrome   p.

Diagnostic Imaging

Best Test(s)
- CT of abdomen with contrast

Ancillary Tests
- Ultrasound of abdomen is useful in young women and children

Lab Evaluation

Best Test(s)
- Gram stain and culture and sensitivity (C&S) of abscess

Ancillary Tests
- CBC with differential
- Blood culture × 2
- ALT, AST
- BUN, creatinine, glucose

Diagnostic Algorithm

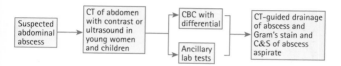

2. Abruptio Placentae

Diagnostic Imaging

Best Test(s)
- Obstetric ultrasound

Ancillary Tests
- Continuous fetal heart rate monitoring

Lab Evaluation

Best Test(s)
- None

Ancillary Tests
- CBC (to quantify blood loss)
- Coagulation profile (PT, PTT, platelets, fibrinogen)
- Blood type and antibody screen to identify Rh-negative patients who may need Rh immunoglobulin

Diagnostic Algorithm

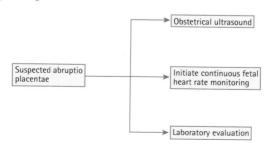

Diagnostic Imaging

Best Test(s)
• Barium swallow with fluoroscopy

Ancillary Tests
• Esophageal manometry if barium swallow is inconclusive
• Upper endoscopy

Lab Evaluation

Best Test(s)
• None

Ancillary Tests
• CBC
• Serum albumin for nutritional assessment

Diagnostic Algorithm

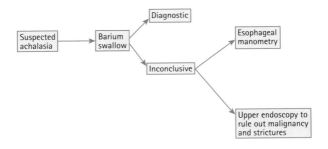

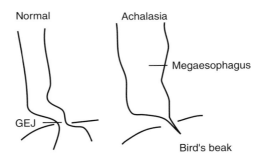

Figure 3-1 Achalasia. *(From Weissleder R, Wittenberg J, Harisinghani MG, Chen JW: Primer of Diagnostic Imaging, ed 4, St. Louis, Mosby, 2007.)*

Diagnostic Imaging

Best Test(s)
• MRI with gadolinium of brain and auditory canal

Ancillary Tests
• CT of brain and auditory canal with IV contrast if MRI is contraindicated

Lab Evaluation

Best Test(s)
• None

Ancillary Tests
• None

Diagnostic Algorithm

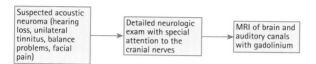

---

5. Acquired Immunodeficiency Syndrome

Diagnostic Imaging

Best Test(s)
• None

Ancillary Tests
• MRI or CT of brain for encephalopathy or focal CNS complications
• Pulmonary gallium scan in suspected *Pneumocystis* pneumonia

Lab Evaluation

Best Test(s)
• HIV antibody test

Ancillary Tests
• T-lymphocyte subset analysis to determine degree of immunodeficiency
• Viral load assay to plan long-term antiviral therapy

Diagnostic Algorithm

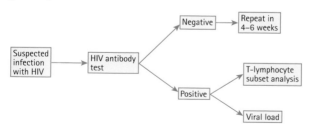

Diagnostic Imaging

Best Test(s)
• MRI of pituitary and hypothalamus with contrast

Ancillary Tests
• CT of pituitary and hypothalamus if MRI is contraindicated

Lab Evaluation

Best Test(s)
• Serum insulin-like growth factor (IGF)-I level

Ancillary Tests
• Suppression test with oral glucose
• Serum phosphate (increased)
• Serum calcium (increased)

Diagnostic Algorithm

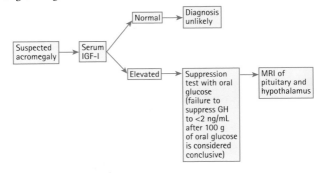

7.   Actinomycosis

Diagnostic Imaging

Best Test(s)
• Chest radiograph

Ancillary Tests
• CT of head, chest, abdomen, and pelvis

Lab Evaluation

Best Test(s)
• Isolation of "sulfur granules" (nests of *Actinomyces* species) from tissue specimens or draining sinuses

Ancillary Tests
• CBC

Diagnostic Algorithm

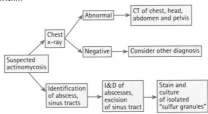

Diagnostic Imaging

Best Test(s)
• Chest radiograph

Ancillary Tests
• CT of chest when lymphangitic carcinomatosis is suspected

Lab Evaluation

Best Test(s)
• ABGs

Ancillary Tests
• CBC with differential
• Blood and urine cultures
• Bronchoalveolar lavage (in selected patients who respond poorly to therapy)

Diagnostic Algorithm

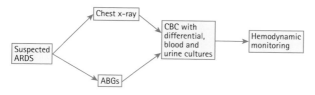

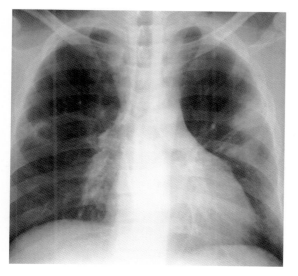

Figure 3-2 ARDS due to extrapulmonary disease. Chest radiograph 2½ days after postoperative hemorrhage. There is diffuse ground-glass opacification, slightly greater on the right than the left. For unknown reasons, the left apex is spared. Incidentally noted are signs of barotraumas—pneumomediastinum and subcutaneous air in the neck. (*From Grainger RG, Allison DJ, Adam A, Dixon AK, eds: Grainger & Allison's Diagnostic Radiology, ed 4, Churchill Livingstone, Philadelphia, 2001.*)

Diagnostic Imaging

Best Test(s)
• None

Ancillary Tests
• CT or MRI of adrenals with contrast
• Chest X-ray

Lab Evaluation

Best Test(s)
• IV cosyntropin test, serial measurement of cortisol

Ancillary Tests
• Serum electrolytes (hyponatremia, hyperkalemia)
• FBS, BUN, creatinine
• CBC (anemia)

Diagnostic Algorithm

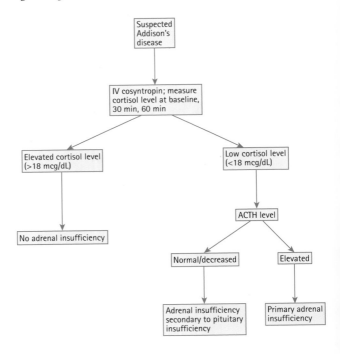

Diagnostic Imaging

Best Test(s)
• MRI of adrenal gland with contrast

Ancillary Tests
• CT of adrenal gland with and without contrast if MRI is contraindicated

Lab Evaluation

Best Test(s)
• Serum electrolytes

Ancillary Tests
• If symptoms of pheochromocytoma, obtain plasma-free metanephrine level, 24-hour urine collection for metanephrines
• If cushingoid appearance, obtain overnight dexamethasone suppression test
• If signs of virilization or feminization, order 24-hour urine for 17-ketosteroids and plasma dehydroepiandrosterone sulfate (DHEAS)
• If hypertension is present with associated hypokalemia, evaluate for aldosteronism

Diagnostic Algorithm

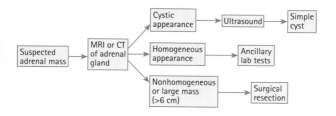

Diagnostic Imaging

Best Test(s)
- None

Ancillary Tests
- MRI with contrast or CT scan of adrenals with contrast to localize neoplasm
- Adrenal scan with iodocholesterol (NP-59) or 6-beta-iodomethyl-19-norcholesterol

Lab Evaluation

Best Test(s)
- Plasma aldosterone concentration (PAC)
- Plasma renin activity (PRA)

Ancillary Tests
- Serum electrolytes
- Aldosterone suppression test

Diagnostic Algorithm

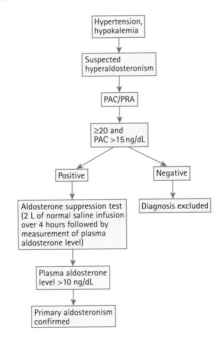

Diagnostic Imaging

Best Test(s)
• CT of liver

Ancillary Tests
• Ultrasound of liver
• Radiograph of pelvis or Paget's disease of bone is suspected

Lab Evaluation

Best Test(s)
• GGT

Ancillary Tests
• Serum calcium, phosphate
• ALT, AST

Diagnostic Algorithm

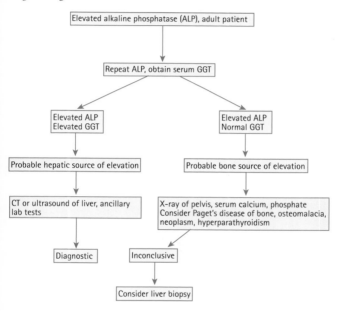

Diagnostic Imaging

Best Test(s)
• None

Ancillary Tests
• Chest radiograph (usually reveals emphysematous changes)

Lab Evaluation

Best Test(s)
• Serum protein alpha$_1$-antitrypsin level

Ancillary Tests
• Pulmonary function tests (PFTs)
• C-reactive protein (CRP)

Diagnostic Algorithm

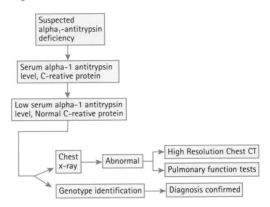

Diagnostic Imaging

Best Test(s)
• CT of liver

Ancillary Tests
• Ultrasound of liver

Lab Evaluation

Best Test(s)
• None

Ancillary Tests
• Ferritin/transferrin saturation
• Viral hepatitis serology
• GGT, alkaline phosphatase, bilirubin
• Antimitochondrial antibody (AMA),
  anti–smooth muscle antibody
  (ASMA), antinuclear antibody (ANA)

Diagnostic Algorithm

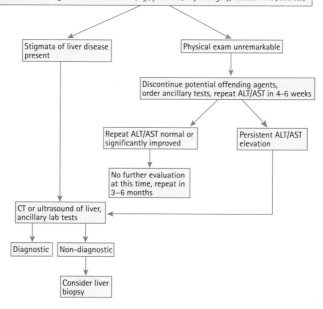

Diagnostic Imaging

Best Test(s)
• None

Ancillary Tests
• PET scan or HMPAO SPECT of brain (selected cases only)
• CT or MRI of brain to rule out (r/o) hydrocephalus or mass lesion and document atrophy (selected cases)

Lab Evaluation

Best Test(s)
• None

Ancillary Tests
• TSH, B_{12} level, methylmalonic acid
• VDRL, HIV (selected patients)
• Basic metabolic profile

Diagnostic Algorithm

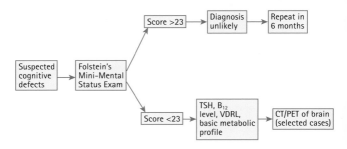

Diagnostic Imaging

Best Test(s)
- Carotid Doppler is best initial test

Ancillary Tests
- MRA of cerebral circulation
- Echocardiogram (r/o embolic source)
- MRI of brain with diffusion-weighted imaging (P/O INFARCT)

Lab Evaluation

Best Test(s)
- Lipid panel
- ESR (r/o temporal arteritis)

Ancillary Tests
- CBC
- PT, PTT, platelet count
- VDRL, toxicology (based on patient's history and age)
- Coagulopathy screening in young patient or with family history (hx) of coagulopathy (e.g., protein C, protein S, anticardiolipin Ab, fibrinogen level)
- ANA

Diagnostic Algorithm

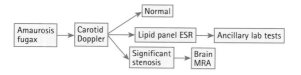

---

17. Amebiasis

Diagnostic Imaging

Best Test(s)
- CT of liver with IV contrast when amebic abscess is suspected

Ancillary Tests
- Ultrasound of liver if CT not readily available

Lab Evaluation

Best Test(s)
- Stool exam for ova and parasites (O&P)

Ancillary Tests
- Serum antibody for *Entamoeba histolytica*

Diagnostic Algorithm

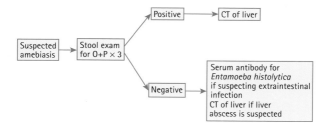

Diagnostic Imaging

Best Test(s)
• MRI of pituitary/hypothalamus with gadolinium when hypothalamic/pituitary lesion is suspected

Ancillary Tests
• Pelvic ultrasound

Lab Evaluation

Best Test(s)
• FSH
• Prolactin
• TSH

Ancillary Tests
• Serum hCG

Diagnostic Algorithm

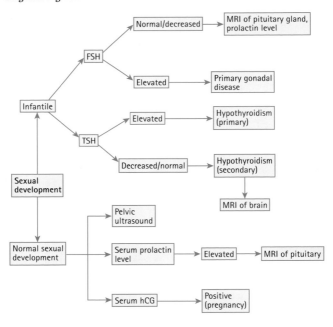

Diagnostic Imaging

Best Test(s)
• MRI of pituitary/hypothalamus with gadolinium when hypothalamic/pituitary lesion is suspected

Ancillary Tests
• Pelvic ultrasound
• CT or MRI of adrenals

Lab Evaluation

Best Test(s)
• Serum hCG
• Prolactin
• FSH

Ancillary Tests
• LH
• Testosterone, DHEAS
• TSH

Diagnostic Algorithm

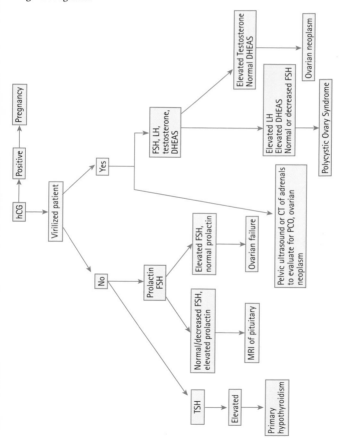

Diagnostic Imaging

Best Test(s)
• None

Ancillary Tests
• Chest radiograph
• Echocardiogram
• Serum amyloid P scintigraphy

Lab Evaluation

Best Test(s)
• Subcutaneous fat aspiration and Congo red staining
• Rectal biopsy (positive in $> 60\%$ of cases) to demonstrate amyloid deposits in tissue

Ancillary Tests
• Serum and urine immunoelectrophoresis (IEP)
• CBC, TSH, creatinine, ALT
• Urinalysis

Diagnostic Algorithm

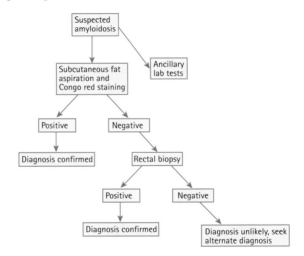

Diagnostic Imaging

Best Test(s)
• None

Ancillary Tests
• Chest radiograph
• MRI of brain and spinal cord
• Modified Barium swallow to evaluate aspiration risk

Lab Evaluation

Best Test(s)
• None

Ancillary Tests
• Lumbar puncture (LP) and CSF analysis
• B_{12} level, TSH, HIV, lead level
• Serum protein IEP
• Muscle biopsy in selected patients to rule out myopathy

Diagnostic Algorithm

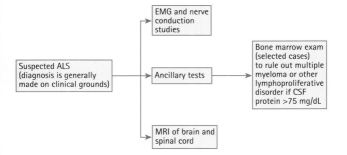

Diagnostic Imaging

Best Test(s)
• None

Ancillary Tests
• None

Lab Evaluation

Best Test(s)
• Reticulocyte count

Ancillary Tests
• Serum B$_{12}$ level, RBC folate level
• ALT, AST, gammaglutamyl
  transpeptidase (GGTP)
• TSH

Diagnostic Algorithm

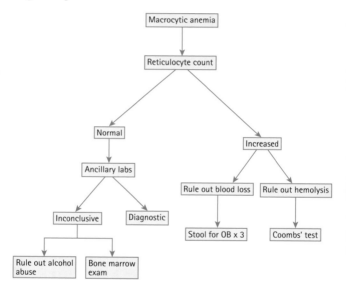

Diagnostic Imaging

Best Test(s)
• None

Ancillary Tests
• None

Lab Evaluation

Best Test(s)
• Reticulocyte count
• Stool for occult blood test × 3

Ancillary Tests
• Ferritin level
• TIBC, serum iron
• Hemoglobin electrophoresis
• Serum lead level

Diagnostic Algorithm

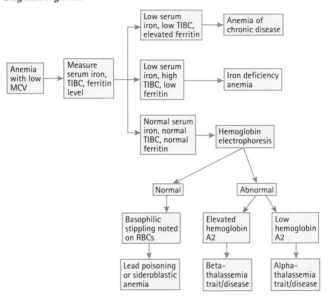

Diagnostic Imaging

Best Test(s)
- Ultrasound of abdominal aorta is best *initial* screening test; CT is more accurate test

Ancillary Tests
- CT of abdominal aorta with IV contrast for preoperative imaging and size estimation and to diagnose perforation/tear
- Angiography for detailed arterial anatomy before surgery

Lab Evaluation

Best Test(s)
- None

Ancillary Tests
- None

Diagnostic Algorithm

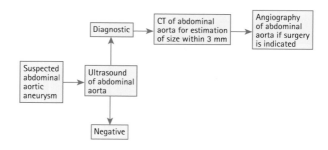

Diagnostic Imaging

Best Test(s)
• None

Ancillary Tests
• None

Lab Evaluation

Best Test(s)
• ANA pattern evaluation

Ancillary Tests
• Anti-Ds DNA Ab
• Anti-Smith Ab
• Anti-RNP Ab
• Anti-SS-A, Anti-SS-B
• ESR
• CBC

Diagnostic Algorithm

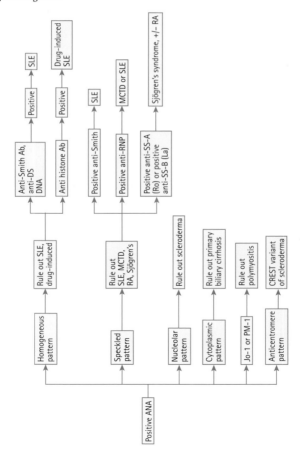

Diagnostic Imaging

Best Test(s)
• None

Ancillary Tests
• Ultrasound in suspected deep vein thrombosis (DVT)
• MRI or CT of brain in patient with neurologic symptoms

Lab Evaluation

Best Test(s)
• Anticardiolipin Ab by ELISA
• Lupus anticoagulant

Ancillary Tests
• ANA
• PT, PTT, platelet count
• VDRL, CBC
• Protein C, protein S, antithrombin III level, factor V Leiden, factor VIII, factor XI, homocysteine level

Diagnostic Algorithm

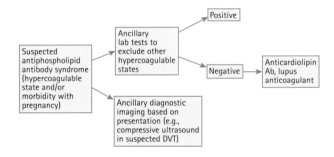

Diagnostic Imaging

Best Test(s)
- CT (sensitivity 83%-100%); CT of aorta is generally readily available and performed as the initial diagnostic modality in suspected aortic dissection

Ancillary Tests
- MRI (sensitivity 90%-100%); difficult test for unstable, intubated patient
- TEE (sensitivity 97%-100%); can also detect aortic insufficiency and pericardial effusion
- Aortography (sensitivity 80%-90%); involves IV contrast; allows visualization of coronary arteries
- Chest radiograph, ECG

Lab Evaluation

Best Test(s)
- None

Ancillary Tests
- CBC
- BUN, creatinine

Diagnostic Algorithm

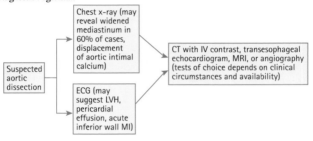

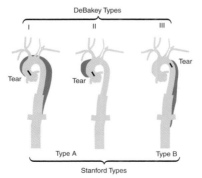

Figure 3-3 Aortic dissection. *(From Weissleder R, Wittenberg J, Harisinghani MG, Chen JW: Primer of Diagnostic Imaging, ed 4, St. Louis, Mosby, 2007.)*

Diagnostic Imaging

Best Test(s)
- CT of appendix with oral and IV contrast

Ancillary Tests
- Ultrasound of pelvis may be used instead of CT in children and/or women of reproductive age when CT is unavailable or contraindicated

Lab Evaluation

Best Test(s)
- CBC with differential
- Urinalysis

Ancillary Tests
- Serum pregnancy test in women of reproductive age

Diagnostic Algorithm

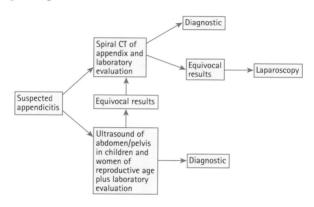

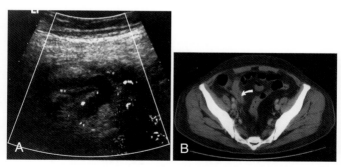

Figure 3-4 Appendicitis. **A,** Ultrasound shows a thickened hypoechoic tubular blind-ended structure in the right iliac fossa. The surrounding fat is hyperchoic. **B,** CT shows the thickened inflamed appendix *(arrow)*. (Courtesy of Dr. A McLean, St. Bartholomew's Hospital, London. From Grainger RG, Allison DJ, Adam A, Dixon AK, eds: *Grainger & Allison's Diagnostic Radiology,* ed 4, Churchill Livingstone, Philadelphia, 2001.)

Diagnostic Imaging

Best Test(s)
- Plain radiograph of affected joint to r/o fracture, neoplasm, destruction of adjacent bone is best initial test

Ancillary Tests
- CT with contrast for early diagnosis in suspected infection of spine, hips, or sternoclavicular and sacroiliac joints

Lab Evaluation

Best Test(s)
- Joint aspiration, Gram stain and C&S of synovial fluid (gonococcal culture if GC is suspected clinically)

Ancillary Tests
- CBC with differential
- Blood culture × 2
- ESR (nonspecific)
- Uric acid
- Lyme titer (in endemic areas)
- Examination of joint fluid for crystals (uric acid, calcium pyrophosphate)

Diagnostic Algorithm

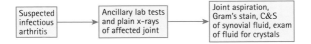

Suspected infectious arthritis → Ancillary lab tests and plain x-rays of affected joint → Joint aspiration, Gram's stain, C&S of synovial fluid, exam of fluid for crystals

Diagnostic Imaging

Best Test(s)
• None

Ancillary Tests
• Chest radiograph (may reveal oval or round infiltrates [Löffler's syndrome])
• Plain films of abdomen and contrast studies (small bowel series) may reveal worm masses in loops of bowel
• Ultrasound and ERCP when worms in pancreatobiliary tract are suspected

Lab Evaluation

Best Test(s)
• Examination of stool for *Ascaris* ova
• *Ascaris* IG4 antibody by ELISA

Ancillary Tests
• Eosinophil count
• CBC
• ALT, AST

Diagnostic Algorithm

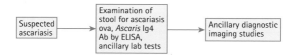

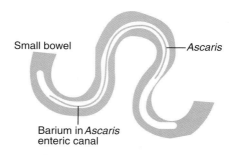

Small bowel — Ascaris

Barium in *Ascaris* enteric canal

Figure 3-5 Ascariasis. *(From Weissleder R, Wittenberg J, Harisinghani MG, Chen JW: Primer of Diagnostic Imaging, ed 4, St. Louis, Mosby, 2007.)*

Diagnostic Imaging

Best Test(s)
• Ultrasound of abdomen/pelvis is best initial diagnostic test

Ancillary Tests
• CT of abdomen/pelvis

Lab Evaluation

Best Test(s)
• Analysis of paracentesis fluid for LDH, glucose, albumin, total protein

Ancillary Tests
• Paracentesis fluid analysis for cell count and differential, Gram stain, AFB stain, bacterial and fungal cultures, amylase
• Serum LDH, protein, albumin
• CBC, ALT, AST, BUN, creative

Diagnostic Algorithm

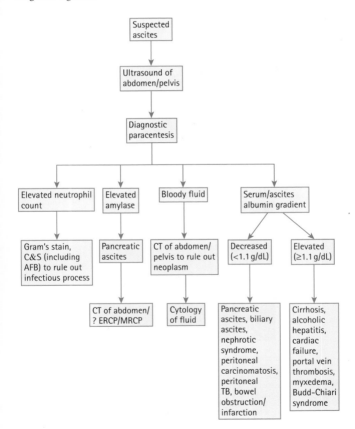

Diagnostic Imaging

Best Test(s)
• MRI of affected joint

Ancillary Tests
• Bone scan if MRI is contraindicated or not readily available
• Plain films of affected joint usually insensitive in early course

Lab Evaluation

Best Test(s)
• None

Ancillary Tests
• CBC with differential
• ESR (nonspecific)
• ANA

Diagnostic Algorithm

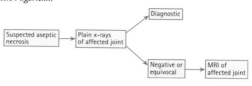

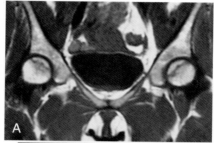

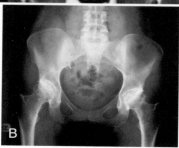

Figure 3-6 Aseptic necrosis of the hip in a renal transplant recipient. **A,** Early changes consisting of low intensity oblique lines are noted by magnetic resonance imaging. **B,** Late changes of AVN by radiograph show narrowing of the hip joint space, sclerosis of the femoral head, and flattening of the left femoral head. *(From Johnson RJ, Feehally J: Comprehensive Clinical Nephrology, ed 2, St. Louis, Mosby, 2000.)*

Diagnostic Imaging

Best Test(s)
• MRI of LS spine

Ancillary Tests
• Plain radiographs of spine
• CT scan of LS spine if MRI is contraindicated
• Ultrasound or CT of abdominal aorta if AAA is suspected

Lab Evaluation

Best Test(s)
• None

Ancillary Tests
• CBC
• ESR
• Urinalysis

Diagnostic Algorithm

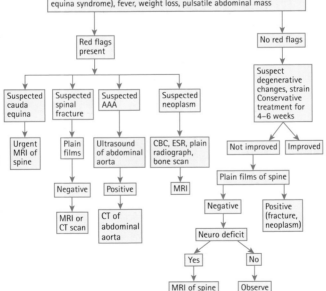

Diagnostic Imaging

Best Test(s)
• Ultrasound of affected lower extremity

Ancillary Tests
• MRI of knee useful preoperatively to
identify coexisting joint pathology

Lab Evaluation

Best Test(s)
• None

Ancillary Tests
• None

Diagnostic Algorithm

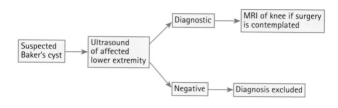

Diagnostic Imaging

Best Test(s)
• None

Ancillary Tests
• Ultrasound of abdomen
• CT of abdomen
• ERCP
• MRCP

Lab Evaluation

Best Test(s)
• Bilirubin fractionation

Ancillary Tests
• Alkaline phosphatase
• ALT, AST, PT (INR)
• CBC
• Coombs' test, haptoglobin
• Hepatitis panel
• ANA
• LDH

Diagnostic Algorithm

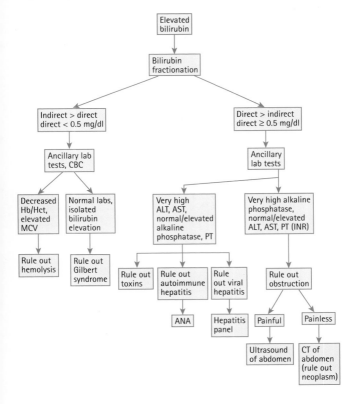

Diagnostic Imaging

Best Test(s)
• None

Ancillary Tests
• None

Lab Evaluation

Best Test(s)
• PT, PTT

Ancillary Tests
• Platelet count
• Clot stability test
• Thrombin time (TT)
• Factor VIII, IX assay
• Bleeding time or platelet function analysis (PFA) 100 assay
• Fibrinogen level
• Factor II, V, X, XIII

Diagnostic Algorithm

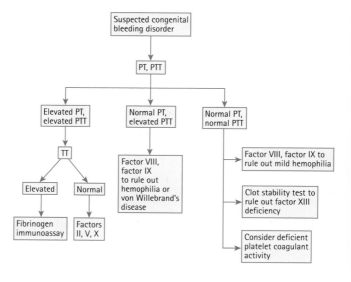

Diagnostic Imaging

Best Test(s)
• MRI of brain with contrast

Ancillary Tests
• CT scan with IV contrast if MRI is contraindicated
• Echocardiography if bacterial endocarditis is suspected source of septic emboli to brain

Lab Evaluation

Best Test(s)
• CBC with differential

Ancillary Tests
• Blood cultures (10% positive)
• ESR

Diagnostic Algorithm

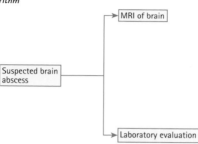

38. Breast Abscess

Diagnostic Imaging

Best Test(s)
• Ultrasound of breast

Ancillary Tests
• None

Lab Evaluation

Best Test(s)
• Gram stain and C&S of abscess contents

Ancillary Tests
• CBC with differential
• Blood cultures

Diagnostic Algorithm

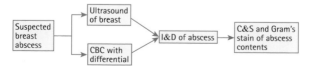

Diagnostic Imaging

Best Test(s)
• MRI of breast without contrast

Ancillary Tests
• Breast ultrasound if MRI is contraindicated

Lab Evaluation

Best Test(s)
• None

Ancillary Tests
• None

Diagnostic Algorithm

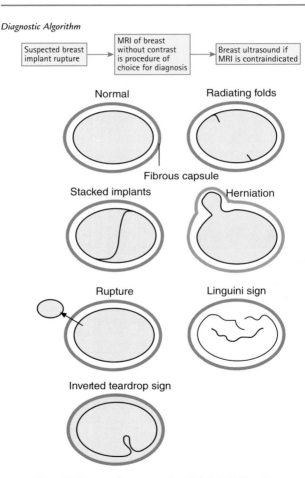

Figure 3-7 Breast implant rupture. *(From Weissleder R, Wittenberg J, Harisinghani MG, Chen JW: Primer of Diagnostic Imaging, ed 4, St. Louis, Mosby, 2007.)*

Diagnostic Imaging

Best Test(s)
- Diagnostic mammogram
- Breast ultrasound

Ancillary Tests
- MRI of breast in selected cases (e.g., breast implant)

Lab Evaluation

Best Test(s)
- None

Ancillary Tests
- Aspiration and cytology of breast cyst

Diagnostic Algorithm

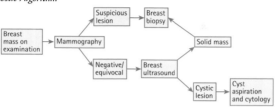

---

41. Breast Nipple Discharge

Diagnostic Imaging

Best Test(s)
- Mammogram

Ancillary Tests
- Ultrasound of breast
- Galactogram
- Breast MRI

Lab Evaluation

Best Test(s)
- Prolactin level

Ancillary Tests
- TSH

Diagnostic Algorithm

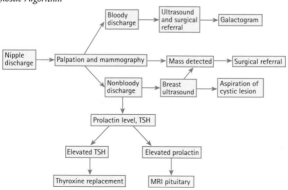

Diagnostic Imaging

Best Test(s)
- Noncontrast high-resolution CT of chest (use of 1- to 1.5-mm window for every 1 cm of acquisition)

Ancillary Tests
- Chest anteroposterior (PA) radiograph (usually reveals hyperventilation, crowded lung markings, small cystic spaces at base of lungs)

Lab Evaluation

Best Test(s)
- None

Ancillary Tests
- Sputum Gram stain, C&S, AFB stain and culture
- CBC with differential
- Serum protein IEP (r/o hypogamma-globulinemia)
- Purified protein derivative (PPD)
- Serum antibody test for aspergillosis
- Sweat test (Pilocarpine intophosesis) in patients with suspected cystic fibrosis

Diagnostic Algorithm

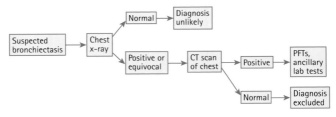

Diagnostic Imaging

Best Test(s)
• Doppler ultrasound of abdomen

Ancillary Tests
• MRI or CT scan of abdomen with IV contrast (may demonstrate collateral circulation and poor visualization of hepatic veins)
• TC-99SC scintigraphy (may demonstrate uptake in the region of the caudate lobe in patients with hepatic vein thrombus)

Lab Evaluation

Best Test(s)
• None

Ancillary Tests
• ALT, AST, alkaline phosphatase
• Bilirubin, platelet count
• Viral hepatitis panel
• ANA, alpha$_1$-antitrypsin level, ceruloplasmin level, anti–smooth muscle Ab, antimitochondrial Ab
• Toxicology screen

Diagnostic Algorithm

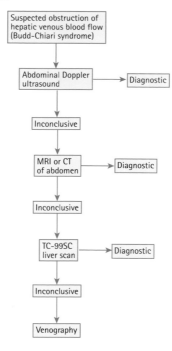

Diagnostic Imaging

Best Test(s)
• CT scan of abdomen, pelvis, and chest with oral and IV contrast to localize tumor and detect metastases

Ancillary Tests
• Echocardiogram or cardiac MRI in suspected cardiac carcinoid
• Radionuclide iodine-113–labeled somatostatin scan (123-ISS) (octreotide scan)

Lab Evaluation

Best Test(s)
• 24-hour urine for HIAA

Ancillary Tests
• ALT, AST
• Serum electrolytes, BUN, creatinine
• Alkaline phosphatase

Diagnostic Algorithm

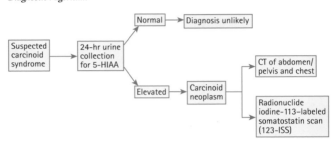

Diagnostic Imaging

Best Test(s)
• Echocardiogram

Ancillary Tests
• Cardiac MRI if pericardial thickening
  or mass
• ECG

Lab Evaluation

Best Test(s)
• None

Ancillary Tests
• TSH
• Creatinine, ALT
• ESR

Diagnostic Algorithm

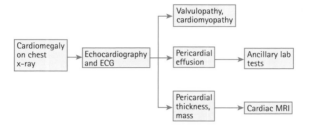

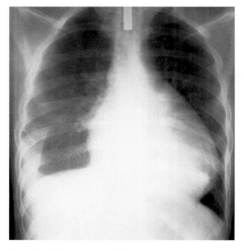

Figure 3-8 Chest radiograph from a patient with a pericardial effusion showing typical "water bottle" heart. *(From Crawford MH, DiMarco JP, Paulus WJ, eds: Cardiology, ed 2, St. Louis, Mosby, 2004.)*

Diagnostic Imaging

Best Test(s)
• None

Ancillary Tests
• None

Lab Evaluation

Best Test(s)
• Culture of lymphatic aspirate
• Biopsy of enlarged lymph node (Warthin-Starry silver stain used to identify bacillus)

Ancillary Tests
• Cat-scratch disease (CSD) skin test
• CBC with differential
• ESR (nonspecific)
• LP in patients with neurologic manifestations

Diagnostic Algorithm

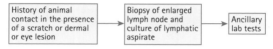

47.   Cavernous Sinus Thrombosis

Diagnostic Imaging

Best Test(s)
• MRI of cavernous sinus with magnetic resonance venography (MRV)

Ancillary Tests
• CT of sinuses can be used to differentiate sphenoid sinusitis from cavernous sinus thrombosis and may also reveal source of thrombosis

Lab Evaluation

Best Test(s)
• None

Ancillary Tests
• CBC with differential
• ESR (nonspecific)
• Blood culture × 2
• Sinus cultures
• LP to r/o meningitis

Diagnostic Algorithm

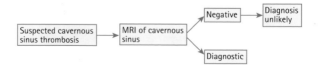

Diagnostic Imaging

Best Test(s)
• None

Ancillary Tests
• Small-bowel series
• Upper endoscopy with biopsy of duodenum/proximal jejunum
• Capsule endoscopy

Lab Evaluation

Best Test(s)
• IgA endomysial Ab is best screening test
• Antigliadin Ab (elevated in > 90% of patients)

Ancillary Tests
• CBC, B_{12} level, folate level
• Serum magnesium, calcium, albumin

Diagnostic Algorithm

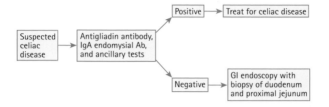

Diagnostic Imaging

Best Test(s)
- CT of head without contrast initially, repeated subsequently with contrast
- MRI of brain can be substituted for CT with contrast

Ancillary Tests
- Carotid Doppler ultrasound
- Echocardiogram

Lab Evaluation

Best Test(s)
- None

Ancillary Tests
- PT, PTT, platelet count
- Lipid panel, glucose
- ALT, electrolytes, BUN, creatinine
- CBC

Diagnostic Algorithm

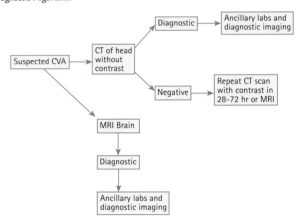

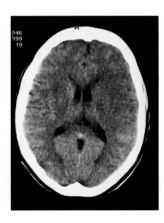

Figure 3-9 Acute ischaemic infarct in the left cerebral artery territory. **A,** CT less than 24 hours from onset of stroke shows loss of gray–white-matter differentiation in the left frontal region and obscuration of the caudate and lentiform nuclei. There is effacement of the left frontal sulci. **B,** At 48 hours the infarct is well defined and exerts more mass effect. *(From Grainger RG, Allison DJ, Adam A, Dixon AK, eds: Grainger & Allison's Diagnostic Radiology, ed 4, Churchill Livingstone, Philadelphia, 2001.)*

Diagnostic Imaging

Best Test(s)
- Ultrasound of abdomen is preferred initial screening test; allows visualization of gallbladder and bile ducts to differentiate extrahepatic obstruction from intrahepatic cholestasis; insensitive but specific for visualization of common duct stones

Ancillary Tests
- CT of abdomen is less accurate for gallstones but more sensitive than ultrasound for visualization of bilirubin distal part of common bile duct; also allows better definition of neoplasm
- ERCP indicated if CT or ultrasound is inconclusive; confirms obstruction and its level, allows collection of specimen for culture and cytology, and provides relief of obstruction
- MRCP can be used to visualize common bile duct and level of obstruction

Lab Evaluation

Best Test(s)
- CBC with differential
- Blood culture × 2

Ancillary Tests
- Serum amylase, lipase
- ALT, AST, alkaline phosphatase

Diagnostic Algorithm

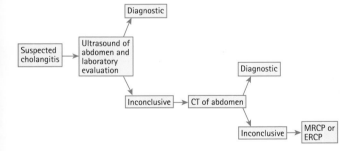

Diagnostic Imaging

Best Test(s)
• Ultrasound of gallbladder

Ancillary Tests
• Nuclear imaging (HIDA) scan is useful for suspected acalculous cholecystitis or when ultrasound is inconclusive
• CT of abdomen useful in suspected abscess, neoplasm, or pancreatitis

Lab Evaluation

Best Test(s)
• CBC with differential

Ancillary Tests
• Alkaline phosphatase
• ALT, AST, bilirubin
• Serum amylase

Diagnostic Algorithm

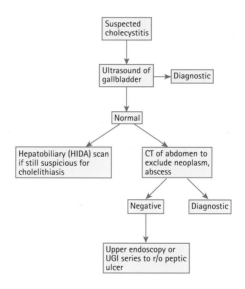

Diagnostic Imaging

Best Test(s)
• Ultrasound of gallbladder will detect stones and biliary sludge (sensitivity 95%, specificity 90%)

Ancillary Tests
• CT of abdomen useful in patients with inconclusive ultrasound to r/o neoplasm or abscess mimicking cholelithiasis; however, it is less sensitive than ultrasound for cholelithiasis

Lab Evaluation

Best Test(s)
• None

Ancillary Tests
• Lipid panel
• ALT, alkaline phosphatase, bilirubin

Diagnostic Algorithm

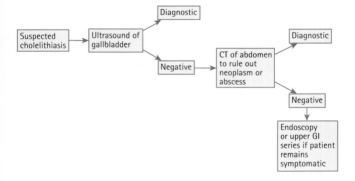

Diagnostic Imaging

Best Test(s)
- Continuous-wave Doppler to measure systolic arterial pressure and ankle-brachial index (ABI)
  Normal ratio of ankle pressure to brachial pressure is 1; in claudication, ABI ranges from 0.5 to 0.8; in patients with rest pain or impending limb loss, ABI is ≤ 0.3

Ancillary Tests
- MRA to locate occluded areas and to assess patency of distal arterial system or previous vein grafts
- Angiography indicated only if surgical reconstruction is being considered

Lab Evaluation

Best Test(s)
- None

Ancillary Tests
- FBS
- Lipid panel
- Creatinine

Diagnostic Algorithm

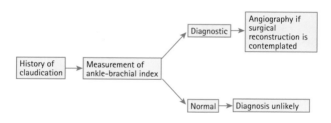

Diagnostic Imaging

Best Test(s)
• None

Ancillary Tests
• Barium enema if patient refuses colonoscopy

Lab Evaluation

Best Test(s)
• None

Ancillary Tests
• CBC
• TSH
• Serum calcium, electrolytes, BUN, creatinine, ALT

Diagnostic Algorithm

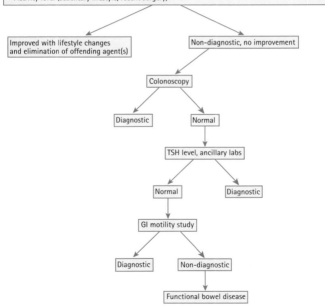

Diagnostic Imaging

Best Test(s)
• None

Ancillary Tests
• None

Lab Evaluation

Best Test(s)
• CPK fractionation

Ancillary Tests
• Serum troponin levels
• CBC, electrolytes, BUN, ALT, creatinine
• TSH, urinalysis

Diagnostic Algorithm

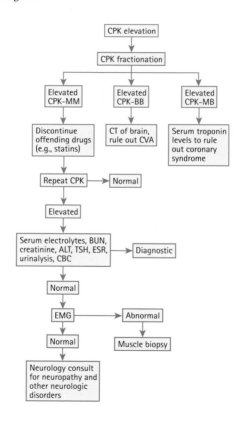

Diagnostic Imaging

Best Test(s)
- MRI or CT of adrenals with IV contrast in suspected adrenal Cushing's syndrome
- MRI of brain with gadolinium in suspected pituitary Cushing's syndrome

Ancillary Tests
- CT of chest in patients with ectopic ACTH production to r/o neoplasm of lung, kidney, or pancreas

Lab Evaluation

Best Test(s)
- Overnight dexamethasone suppression test
- Plasma cortisol

Ancillary Tests
- Electrolytes, creatinine, glucose

Diagnostic Algorithm

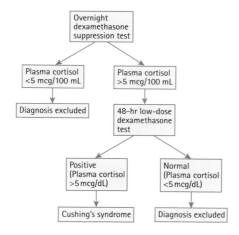

Diagnostic Imaging

Best Test(s)
- Chest radiograph (PA)

Ancillary Tests
- Echocardiogram
- Spiral CT of chest

Lab Evaluation

Best Test(s)
- Arterial blood gases

Ancillary Tests
- ANA, ESR, creatinine, ALT
- CBC, hemoglobin electrophoresis
- Methemoglobin level

Diagnostic Algorithm

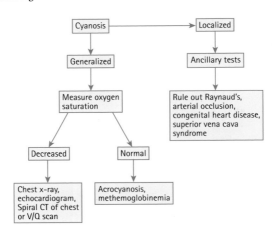

Diagnostic Imaging

Best Test(s)
• Compressive duplex ultrasonography of affected extremity

Ancillary Tests
• Contrast venography; "gold standard" but invasive and painful
• Magnetic resonance direct thrombus imaging (MRDTI); very accurate and noninvasive but limited by cost and availability

Lab Evaluation

Best Test(s)
• D-Dimer assay by ELISA

Ancillary Tests
• PT, PTT, platelet count
• Coagulopathy workup (e.g., protein C, protein S, antithrombin III, factor V Leiden, lupus anticoagulant) in patients with suspected coagulopathy

Diagnostic Algorithm

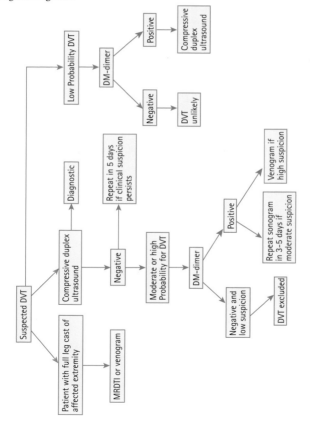

TABLE 3-1 Wells' Clinical Assessment Model For the Pretest Probability of Lower Extremity Deep Vein Thrombosis

	Score
Active cancer (treatment ongoing or within previous 6 months or pallative)	1
Paralysis, paresis or recent plaster immobilization of the lower extremities	1
Recently bedridden > 3 days or major surgery within 4 weeks	1
Localized tenderness along the distribution of the deep venous system	1
Entire leg swollen	1
Calf swelling > 3 cm asymptomatic side (measured 10 cm below tibial tuberosity)	1
Pitting edema confined to the symptomatic leg	1
Collateral superficial veins (nonvaricose)	1
Alternative diagnosis as likely or greater than that of DVT	-2

In patients with symptoms in both legs, the more symptomatic leg is used. Pretest probability is calculated as the total score: high > 3; moderate 1 or 2; low < 0.

From Crawford MH, DiMarco JP, Paulus WJ, eds: *Cardiology,* ed 2, St. Louis, Mosby, 2004.

Diagnostic Imaging

Best Test(s)
• CT of head without contrast to r/o subdural hematoma, hemorrhage

Ancillary Tests
• Chest radiograph

Lab Evaluation

Best Test(s)
• Variable with clinical suspicion and physical examination (e.g., toxicology screen in suspected drug abuse, CSF examination in suspected encephalitis or meningitis, CBC with differential in suspected infectious process)

Ancillary Tests
• Blood culture × 2
• ALT, AST
• TSH, B_{12} level
• BUN, creatinine, urinalysis
• ABGs or pulse oxymetry
• Serum electrolytes, glucose, calcium, phosphate, magnesium

Diagnostic Algorithm

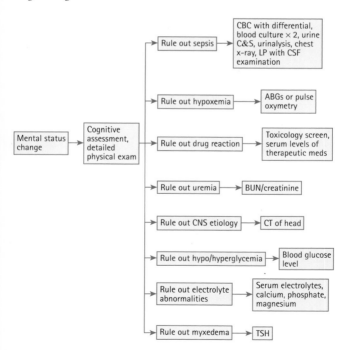

Diagnostic Imaging

Best Test(s)
• None

Ancillary Tests
• MRI of brain with gadolinium if neurogenic diabetes insipidus is confirmed

Lab Evaluation

Best Test(s)
• Water deprivation test

Ancillary Tests
• FBS
• Urinalysis (specific gravity < 1.005; no glycosuria)
• Urine osmolarity (<200mOsm/kg)
• Plasma osmolarity (elevated)
• Serum electrolytes, calcium, BUN, creatinine

Diagnostic Algorithm

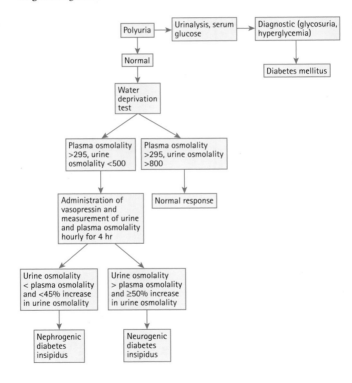

Diagnostic Imaging

Best Test(s)
• None

Ancillary Tests
• Small-bowel series if malabsorption is suspected

Lab Evaluation

Best Test(s)
• Stool for O&P
• Stool for occult blood × 3
• Stool Sudan stain (in malabsorption, mucosal disease, pancreatic insufficiency, bile salt insufficiency)
• Stool osmolality (stool [Na plus K]) × 2

Ancillary Tests
• Serum electrolytes, BUN, creatinine
• Stool Na⁺, K⁺
• CBC with differential
• Stool for *Clostridium difficile* toxin assay
• ALT, AST
• TSH, free T4
• Albumin, total protein, glucose
• Stool cultures for *Escherichia coli, Shigella, Salmonella, Yersinia, Campylobacter, Entamoeba histolytica*
• Antigliadin IgA antibody, endomysial IgA antibody
• Colon biopsy

Diagnostic Algorithm

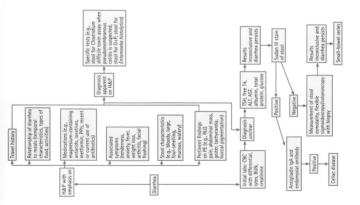

Diagnostic Imaging

Best Test(s)
• None

Ancillary Tests
• Chest radiograph to exclude infectious process in patients presenting with pulmonary symptoms

Lab Evaluation

Best Test(s)
• PT, PTT, Fibrin degradation Products (FDPs), D-dimer, Thrombin time (TT)
• Fibrinogen level, platelets
• CBC, peripheral blood smear

Ancillary Tests
• ALT, AST to r/o liver disease
• Factor V, VIII

Diagnostic Algorithm

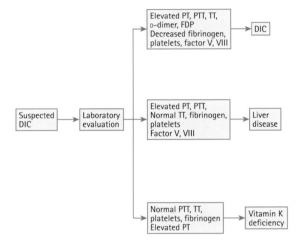

Diagnostic Imaging

Best Test(s)
• CT scan of abdomen and pelvis with oral and IV contrast (typical findings are thickening of bowel wall, abscess formation)

Ancillary Tests
• None

Lab Evaluation

Best Test(s)
• CBC with differential
• Blood culture × 2

Ancillary Tests
• Urinalysis
• ALT, creatinine, BUN, LYTES, Amylase
• Serum pregnancy test in reproductive age female

Diagnostic Algorithm

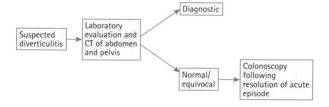

Diagnostic Imaging

Best Test(s)
• None

Ancillary Tests
• UGI series if patient refuses endoscopy
• Chest radiograph

Lab Evaluation

Best Test(s)
• *H. pylori* stool antigen or breath test

Ancillary Tests
• CBC

Diagnostic Algorithm

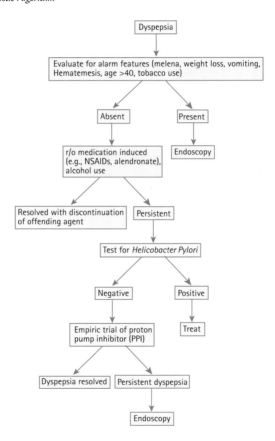

Diagnostic Imaging

Best Test(s)
• Varies with suspected diagnosis

Ancillary Tests
• Upper endoscopy
• Esophageal manometry
• Barium swallow, video swallow

Lab Evaluation

Best Test(s)
• None

Ancillary Tests
• CBC

Diagnostic Algorithm

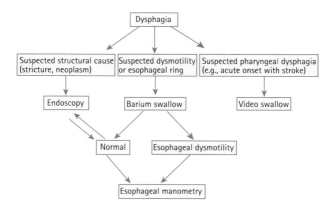

Diagnostic Imaging

Best Test(s)
• Chest radiograph

Ancillary Tests
• ECG
• Echocardiogram
• PFTs
• Helical CT of chest or V/Q scan

Lab Evaluation

Best Test(s)
• CBC (r/o anemia, infection)

Ancillary Tests
• ABGs or pulse oximetry (r/o PE)
• TSH
• Serum electrolytes, BUN, creatinine
• B-type natriuretic peptide (BNP)

Diagnostic Algorithm

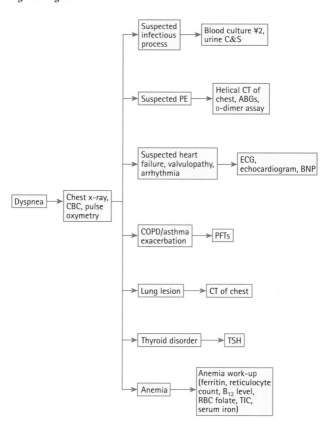

Diagnostic Imaging

Best Test(s)
• None

Ancillary Tests
• Pelvic ultrasound

Lab Evaluation

Best Test(s)
• Gram stain and C&S of urethral discharge
• PCR assay for *Chlamydiae* or *Neisseria gonorrhoe*

Ancillary Tests
• Urinalysis, urine C&S
• VDRL, HIV

Diagnostic Algorithm

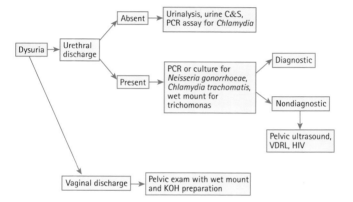

Diagnostic Imaging

Best Test(s)
- CT scan of abdomen and chest with IV contrast

Ancillary Tests
- Ultrasound of abdomen if CT is contraindicated

Lab Evaluation

Best Test(s)
- Histologic examination of cyst or content obtained by aspiration or resection
- *Echinococcus granulosa* hydatid fluid antigen by ELISA

Ancillary Tests
- Echinococcal antibody assay by ELISA and Western blot (>90% sensitive and specific for liver cysts but less accurate for cysts in other sites)

Diagnostic Algorithm

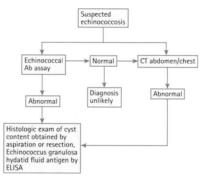

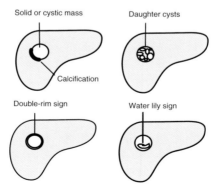

Figure 3-10 Echinococcosis. *(From Weissleder R, Wittenberg J, Harisinghani MG, Chen JW: Primer of Diagnostic Imaging, ed 4, St. Louis, Mosby, 2007.)*

Diagnostic Imaging

Best Test(s)
• Obstetric (transvaginal) ultrasound

Ancillary Tests
• None

Lab Evaluation

Best Test(s)
• Serum hCG (quantitative)

Ancillary Tests
• Serum progesterone (decreased production in ectopic pregnancy)
• CBC
• Urinalysis

Diagnostic Algorithm

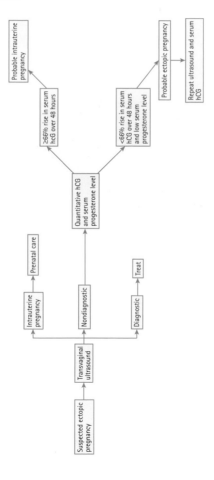

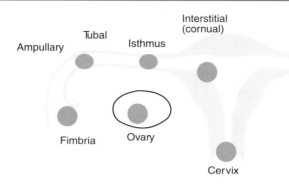

Figure 3-11 Ectopic pregnancy. *(From Weissleder R, Wittenberg J, Harisinghani MG, Chen JW: Primer of Diagnostic Imaging, ed 4, St. Louis, Mosby, 2007.)*

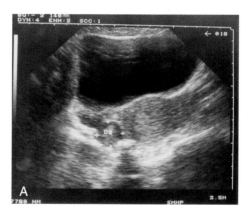

Figure 3-12 Ultrasound scan showing ectopic pregnancy. **A,** Transabdominal scan showing empty uterus with a complex mass in the right adnexa measuring 21 × 22 mm.

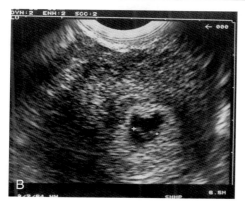

Figure 3-12 **B,** Transvaginal scan showing absence of
gestational sac in the uterus and decidual reaction with
marked endometrial thickening. There is free fluid in the
pouch of Douglas (blood will be found there in ruptured
ectopic pregnancy). *(From Greer IA, Cameron IT, Kitchener
HC, Prentice A: Mosby's Color Atlas and Text of Obstetrics
and Gynecology, London, Harcourt, 2001.)*

Diagnostic Imaging

Best Test(s)
• Chest radiograph

Ancillary Tests
• Echocardiogram
• Abdominal ultrasound

Lab Evaluation

Best Test(s)
• Serum albumin, creatinine
• Urinalysis
• B-type natriuretic peptide (BNP)

Ancillary Tests
• ALT, AST, BUN
• TSH

Diagnostic Algorithm

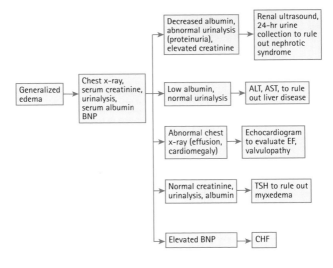

Generalized edema → Chest x-ray, serum creatinine, urinalysis, serum albumin BNP →

- Decreased albumin, abnormal urinalysis (proteinuria), elevated creatinine → Renal ultrasound, 24-hr urine collection to rule out nephrotic syndrome
- Low albumin, normal urinalysis → ALT, AST, to rule out liver disease
- Abnormal chest x-ray (effusion, cardiomegaly) → Echocardiogram to evaluate EF, valvulopathy
- Normal creatinine, urinalysis, albumin → TSH to rule out myxedema
- Elevated BNP → CHF

Diagnostic Imaging

Best Test(s)
- Doppler ultrasound

Ancillary Tests
- Plain x-ray films of extremities in patients with history of musculoskeletal trauma (r/o fracture)
- Echocardiogram (r/o CHF, valvulopathy)
- CT and/or ultrasound of pelvis

Lab Evaluation

Best Test(s)
- None

Ancillary Tests
- D-Dimer by ELISA when DVT is suspected
- Creatinine, ALT, albumin
- TSH
- Urinalysis
- 24-hour urine protein to r/o nephrotic syndrome if urinalysis reveals proteinuria
- BNP

Diagnostic Algorithm

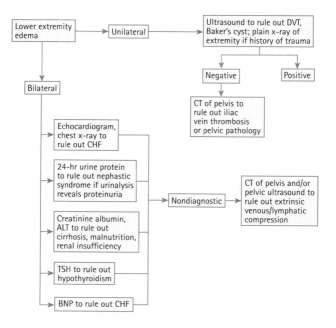

Diagnostic Imaging

Best Test(s)
- Transesophageal echocardiogram (TEE)

Ancillary Tests
- Transthoracic echocardiography if TEE is not readily available or patient is uncooperative

Lab Evaluation

Best Test(s)
- Blood culture × 3

Ancillary Tests
- CBC with differential
- ESR (nonspecific)
- Urinalysis

Diagnostic Algorithm

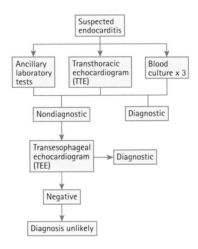

Diagnostic Imaging

Best Test(s)
• None

Ancillary Tests
• Laparoscopy
• Pelvic ultrasound for adnexal mass
• CT or MRI of abdomen/pelvis
• Colonoscopy)

Lab Evaluation

Best Test(s)
• None

Ancillary Tests
• CA 125 (if result > 35U/ml, positive predictive value of 0.58 and negative predictive value of 0.96 for presence of endometriosis)

Diagnostic Algorithm

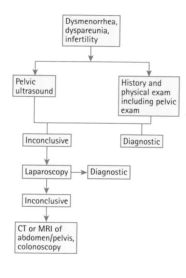

Diagnostic Imaging

Best Test(s)
• None

Ancillary Tests
• CT or ultrasound of kidneys and urinary bladder
• Sleep study
• Urodynamic studies

Lab Evaluation

Best Test(s)
• Urinalysis, urine C&S

Ancillary Tests
• FBS, electrolytes, BUN, creatinine

Diagnostic Algorithm

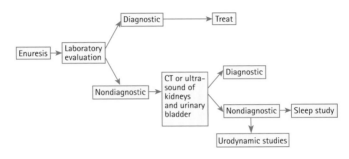

Diagnostic Imaging

Best Test(s)
• Lateral soft tissue radiograph of neck

Ancillary Tests
• Chest radiograph (evidence of pneumonia is present in > 20% of epiglottitis cases)

Lab Evaluation

Best Test(s)
• None

Ancillary Tests
• CBC with differential
• Blood culture × 2
• Culture of epiglottitis (should be obtained only in controlled environment [e.g., OR])

Diagnostic Algorithm

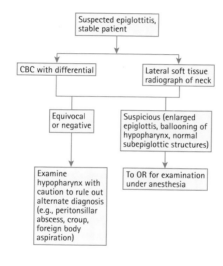

Diagnostic Imaging

Best Test(s)
• Barium swallow

Ancillary Tests
• Chest radiograph (PA and lateral)
• CT of neck and chest

Lab Evaluation

Best Test(s)
• None

Ancillary Tests
• CBC

Diagnostic Algorithm

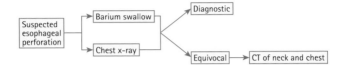

Diagnostic Imaging

Best Test(s)
• None

Ancillary Tests
• Chest radiograph
• ECG
• Polysomnography (sleep study)

Lab Evaluation

Best Test(s)
• CBC with differential

Ancillary Tests
• TSH, B_{12} level
• Electrolytes, BUN, creatinine
• ALT, FBS
• Epstein-Barr (EB) viral titers,
• CMV viral titers
• ESR (nonspecific)

Diagnostic Algorithm

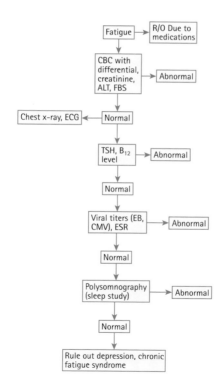

Diagnostic Imaging

Best Test(s)
• None

Ancillary Tests
• Chest radiograph
• Echocardiogram (if blood cultures are positive or SBE suspected clinically)
• CT of chest/abdomen/pelvis

Lab Evaluation

Best Test(s)
• None

Ancillary Tests
• CBC with differential
• Blood culture × 2
• Urinalysis, urine C&S
• ESR, ANA
• ALT, AST, creatinine
• HIV, PPD
• cANCA, pANCA

Diagnostic Algorithm

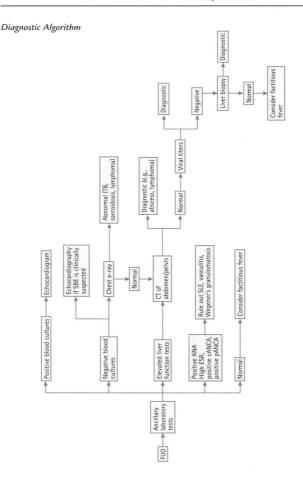

Diagnostic Imaging

Best Test(s)
• None

Ancillary Tests
• None

Lab Evaluation

Best Test(s)
• Variable with appearance of lesion

Ancillary Tests
• VDRL
• Biopsy of lesion
• LGV complement fixation
• *Chlamydia trachomatis* immunofluorescence
• Serology or viral cultures for HSV
• HIV

Diagnostic Algorithm

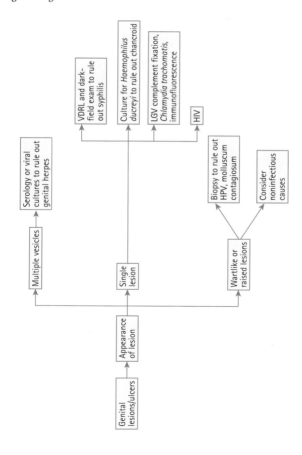

Diagnostic Imaging

Best Test(s)
• Ultrasound of thyroid

Ancillary Tests
• Radioactive iodine uptake (RAIU) scan of thyroid

Lab Evaluation

Best Test(s)
• TSH, free T_4

Ancillary Tests
• CBC with differential
• Antimicrosomal Ab
• Thyroglobulin level

Diagnostic Algorithm

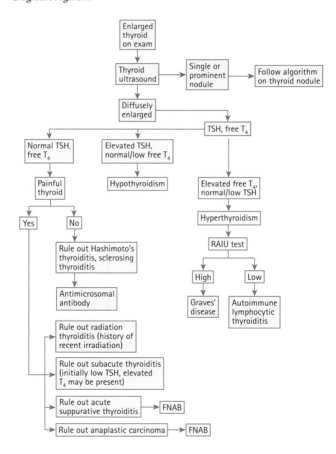

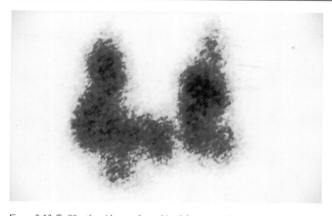

Figure 3-13 Tc-99m thyroid scan of a multinodular goiter. *(From Besser CM, Thorner MO: Comprehensive Clinical Endocrinology, ed 3, St. Louis, Mosby, 2002.)*

81. Gout

Diagnostic Imaging

Best Test(s)
• None

Ancillary Tests
• Plain radiograph of affected joint when diagnosis is unclear

Lab Evaluation

Best Test(s)
• Examination of synovial fluid aspirate from affected joint for presence of urate crystals (needle-shaped and birefringent)

Ancillary Tests
• Serum uric acid level
• CBC with differential, ESR if infectious process is suspected
• Gram stain and C&S of synovial fluid aspirate

Diagnostic Algorithm

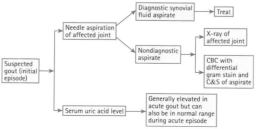

Diagnostic Imaging

Best Test(s)
• None

Ancillary Tests
• Mammography/sonography if unilateral gynecomastia
• MRI of pituitary with contrast if elevated prolactin
• Ultrasound of testicles when testicular lesion is suspected

Lab Evaluation

Best Test(s)
• Serum testosterone, LH
• Prolactin

Ancillary Tests
• ALT, AST, creatinine, urinalysis
• Serum estradiol, hCG

Diagnostic Algorithm

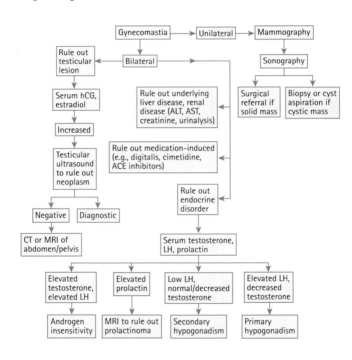

Diagnostic Imaging

Best Test(s)
- None

Ancillary Tests
- CT of head with contrast or MRI with contrast
- CT of temporal bone without contrast

Lab Evaluation

Best Test(s)
- None

Ancillary Tests
- CBC
- ALT, AST
- ANA, VDRL
- TSH

Diagnostic Algorithm

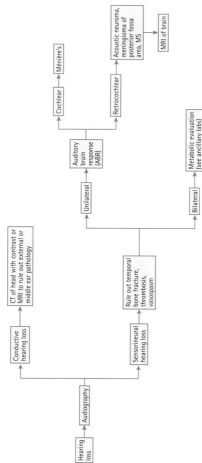

Diagnostic Imaging

Best Test(s)
- Ultrasound of kidneys and urinary bladder

Ancillary Tests
- Spiral CT of abdomen and pelvis without contrast; useful to exclude renal mass and calculi
- IVP (will detect most calculi and papillary necrosis)

Lab Evaluation

Best Test(s)
- Urine microscopy
- Urine C&S

Ancillary Tests
- Urine cytology × 3
- BUN, creatinine
- CBC, platelet count, PT, PTT

Diagnostic Algorithm

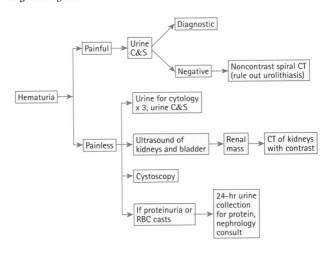

Diagnostic Imaging

Best Test(s)
• None

Ancillary Tests
• Noncontrast CT or MRI of liver; useful for excluding other causes of elevated liver enzymes; imaging of liver may reveal increased density of liver tissue and is also useful in screening for hepatoma (increased risk in patients with cirrhosis)

Lab Evaluation

Best Test(s)
• Plasma transferrin saturation is best screening test
• Plasma ferritin; good indicator of total body iron stores but may be elevated in many other conditions (e.g., inflammation, malignancy)
• Measurement of hepatic iron index (hepatic iron concentration/age) in liver biopsy specimen to confirm diagnosis

Ancillary Tests
• ALT, AST, alkaline phosphatase
• Genetic testing (HFE phenotyping for C282Y and H63D mutations)

Diagnostic Algorithm

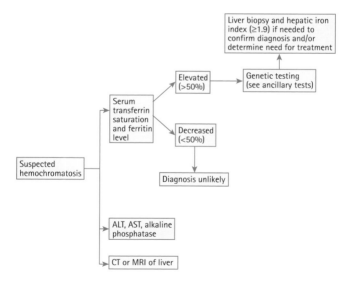

Diagnostic Imaging

Best Test(s)
• None

Ancillary Tests
• None

Lab Evaluation

Best Test(s)
• Factor VIII: C level (decreased in hemophilia A)
• Factor IX coagulant activity level (decreased in hemophilia B)

Ancillary Tests
• PTT (increased), PT (normal)
• Platelet-function analysis (PFA-100 assay), factor VIII antigen, fibrinogen level
• Platelet count, CBC

Diagnostic Algorithm

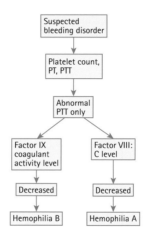

Diagnostic Imaging

Best Test(s)
• Chest radiograph

Ancillary Tests
• Echocardiogram
• Spiral CT of chest

Lab Evaluation

Best Test(s)
• None

Ancillary Tests
• PT, PTT, platelets
• Sputum C&S and Gram stain, AFB stain
• CBC
• ABGs or pulse oxymetry

Diagnostic Algorithm

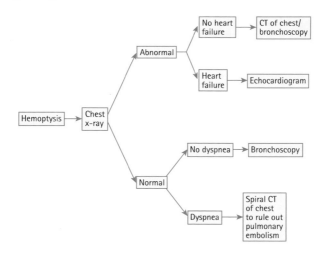

Diagnostic Imaging

Best Test(s)
• None

Ancillary Tests
• Ultrasound of liver or CT in patients with fulminant hepatitis

Lab Evaluation

Best Test(s)
• IgM anti-HAV confirms diagnosis; detectable in almost all infected patients at presentation and remains positive for 3 to 6 months

Ancillary Tests
• IgG anti-HAV may be present at disease onset and peaks 6 to 12 months after the acute illness; may persist for years
• ALT (very elevated), AST (very elevated), alkaline phosphatase (mild elevation), bilirubin (elevated)
• PT (INR) (elevated in severe cases)

Diagnostic Algorithm

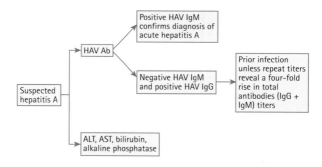

Diagnostic Imaging

Best Test(s)
• None

Ancillary Tests
• Ultrasound or CT of liver in patients who present with fulminant hepatitis

Lab Evaluation

Best Test(s)
• Presence of HBcAb (IgM) confirms either acute or early infection by HBV
• HBsAg is detected in acute or chronic hepatitis B
• HBeAg is marker of acute infection

Ancillary Tests
• ALT (very elevated), AST (very elevated), alkaline phosphatase (mild elevation), bilirubin (elevated)
• PT (INR) in severe cases

Diagnostic Algorithm

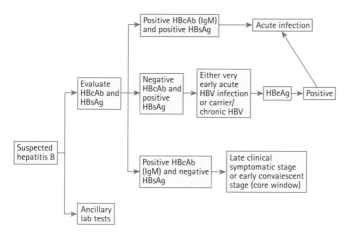

Diagnostic Imaging

Best Test(s)
• None

Ancillary Tests
• Ultrasound or CT of liver in patients who present with fulminant hepatitis or chronic hepatitis C (increased risk of hepato cellular carcinoma)

Lab Evaluation

Best Test(s)
• HCV RNA detects virus as early as 2 to 4 weeks after exposure
• HCV Ab by enzyme immunoassay (EIA) indicates past or present infection but does not differentiate among acute, chronic, or resolved infection; all positive EIA results should be verified with supplemental assay (e.g., recombinant immunoblot assay [RIBA])
• Viral genotyping can distinguish among genotypes 1, 2, 3, and 4 which is helpful in choosing therapy

Ancillary Tests
• ALT (very elevated), AST (very elevated), alkaline phosphatase (mild elevation), bilirubin (elevated)
• PT (INR) in severe cases

Diagnostic Algorithm

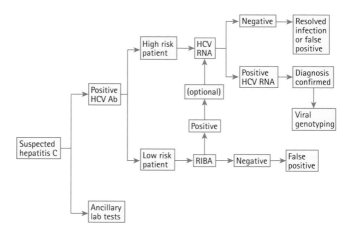

Diagnostic Imaging

Best Test(s)
• CT scan of abdomen

Ancillary Tests
• Ultrasound of abdomen if CT is contraindicated
• Echocardiography if congestive hepatomegaly is suspected

Lab Evaluation

Best Test(s)
• Liver biopsy

Ancillary Tests
• ALT, AST, alkaline phosphatase
• Bilirubin, hepatitis panel, CBC
• FBS, serum albumin, INR
• ANA, AMA, transferrin saturation, ceruloplasmin level, serum copper, alpha-1 antitrypsin level

Diagnostic Algorithm

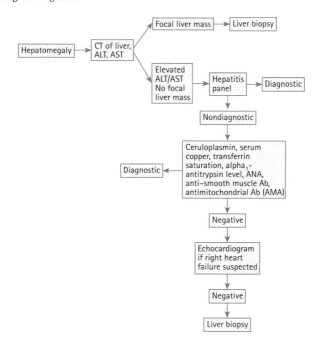

Diagnostic Imaging

Best Test(s)
- None

Ancillary Tests
- Renal ultrasound to r/o obstruction

Lab Evaluation

Best Test(s)
- Calculation of fractional excretion of sodium (FE_{Na}) = [U/P sodium/U/P creatinine] × 100

Ancillary Tests
- Serum electrolytes, creatinine, BUN, osmolality
- Urine sodium, osmolality, creatinine

Diagnostic Algorithm

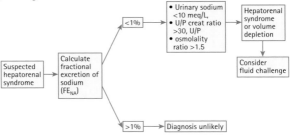

TABLE 3-2 Diagnostic Criteria for Hepatorenal Syndrome

Major Criteria

- Chronic or acute liver disease with advanced hepatic failure and portal hypertension
- Low glomerular filtration rate, as indicated by serum creatinine > 1.5 mg/dl (135 μmol/L) or 24-h creatinine clearance < 40 ml/min
- Absence of shock, ongoing bacterial infection, and current or recent treatment with nephrotoxic drugs
- Absence of gastrointestinal fluid losses (repeated vomiting or intense diarrhea)
- Absence of renal fluid losses (weight loss > 500 g/day for several days in patients with ascites without peripheral edema or 1000 g/day in patients with peripheral edema)
- No sustained improvement in renal function (decrease in serum creatinine to 1.5 mg/dl (135 μmol/L) or less or increase in creatinine clearance to 40 ml/min or more) following diuretic withdrawl and expansion of plasma volume with 1.5 L of isotonic saline
- Proteinuria < 500 mg/day and no ultrasonographic evidence of obstructive uropathy or parenchymal renal disease

Additional Criteria

- Urine volume < 500 ml/day
- Urine sodium < 10 mmol/L
- Urine osmolality greater than plasma osmolality
- Urine red blood cells < 50 per high power field
- Serum sodium concentration < 130 mmol/L

From Johnson RJ, Feehally J: *Comprehensive Clinical Nephrology*, ed 2, St. Louis, Mosby, 2000.

Diagnostic Imaging

Best Test(s)
• None

Ancillary Tests
• CT or MRI of adrenal gland with contrast (R/o adrenal tumors)
• Pelvic ultrasound (R/o ovarian tumor, R/o PCOS)
• MRI of pituitary (R/o pituitary tumor)

Lab Evaluation

Best Test(s)
• Serum testosterone, dehydroepi-androsterone (DS), 17-hydroxypro-gesterone (17-OHP)

Ancillary Tests
• Dexamethasone suppression test
• LH, FSH, FBS

Diagnostic Algorithm

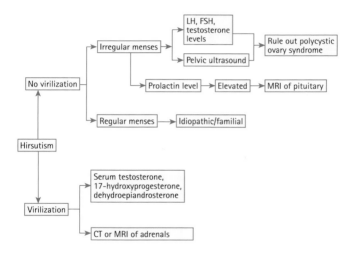

Diagnostic Imaging

Best Test(s)
• MRI of head without contrast

Ancillary Tests
• CT of head without contrast if MRI
  is contraindicated

Lab Evaluation

Best Test(s)
• CSF fluid analysis

Ancillary Tests
• Urinalysis, urine C&S
• FBS

Diagnostic Algorithm

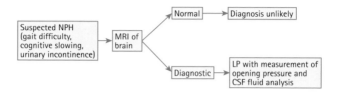

Diagnostic Imaging

Best Test(s)
• None

Ancillary Tests
• Radiograph of painful bones (r/o
  bone neoplasm, multiple myeloma)
• Technetium (Tc) 99m parathyroid
  scan (R/o parathyroid adenoma)
• Ultrasound of parathyroid glands
• Ultrasound of kidneys (R/o renal
  cell carcinoma)

Lab Evaluation

Best Test(s)
• Serum calcium level
• PTH level

Ancillary Tests
• Serum phosphate, magnesium,
  alkaline phosphatase, albumin
• Electrolytes, BUN, creatinine
• 24-hour urine collection for calcium
• Urinary cyclic AMP
• PSA (if prostate carcinoma is
  suspected)
• Serum and urine protein immunoelectrophoresis (if multiple myeloma
  suspected)

Diagnostic Algorithm

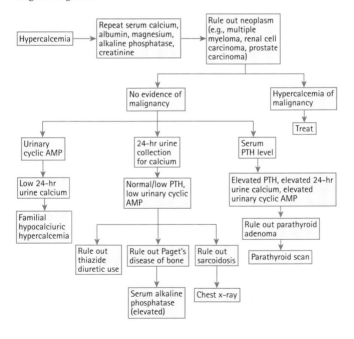

Diagnostic Imaging

Best Test(s)
• None

Ancillary Tests
• None

Lab Evaluation

Best Test(s)
• Heparinized potassium level

Ancillary Tests
• Serum electrolytes, BUN, creatinine
• Glucose, CBC
• CPK (when rhabdomyolysis is suspected)

Diagnostic Algorithm

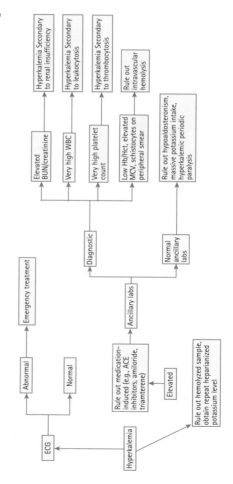

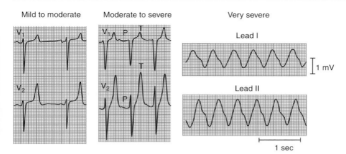

Figure 3-14 The earliest change with hyperkalemia is peaking ("tenting") of the T waves. With progressive increases in serum potassium, the QRS complexes widen, the P waves decrease in amplitude and may disappear, and finally, a sine-wave pattern leads to asystole. *(From Goldberger AL, ed: Clinical Electrocardiography, ed 6, St. Louis, Mosby, 1999.)*

Diagnostic Imaging

Best Test(s)
• None

Ancillary Tests
• None

Lab Evaluation

Best Test(s)
• 24-hour urine magnesium level

Ancillary Tests
• Serum electrolytes, calcium
• BUN, creatinine, glucose
• TSH
• CPK

Diagnostic Algorithm

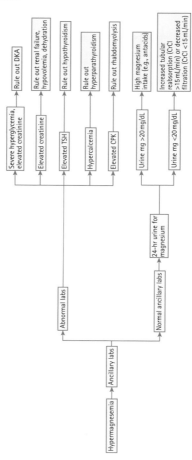

Diagnostic Imaging

Best Test(s)
• None

Ancillary Tests
• None

Lab Evaluation

Best Test(s)
• Serum electrolytes

Ancillary Tests
• Urine sodium, urine osmolality
• BUN, creatinine

Diagnostic Algorithm

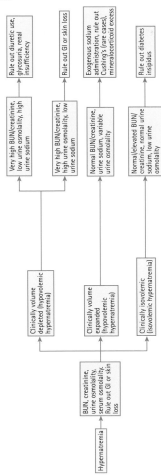

Diagnostic Imaging

Best Test(s)
• None

Ancillary Tests
• None

Lab Evaluation

Best Test(s)
• 24-hour urine phosphate collection

Ancillary Tests
• Serum electrolytes, BUN, creatinine, magnesium, calcium, glucose
• Urinalysis, CPK

Diagnostic Algorithm

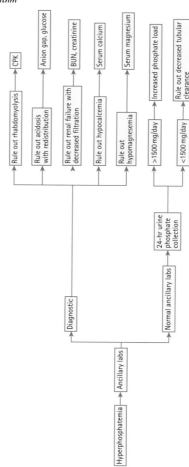

Diagnostic Imaging

Best Test(s)
• None

Ancillary Tests
• Thyroid ultrasound
• RAIU thyroid scan

Lab Evaluation

Best Test(s)
• Free T_4
• TSH

Ancillary Tests
• Free T_3
• Serum thyroglobulin level
• Serum antimicrosomal antibodies

Diagnostic Algorithm

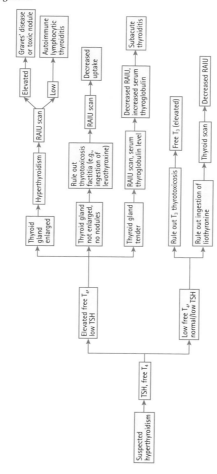

Diagnostic Imaging

Best Test(s)
• None

Ancillary Tests
• None

Lab Evaluation

Best Test(s)
• PTH

Ancillary Tests
• Serum albumin level
• Serum phosphate, magnesium level

Diagnostic Algorithm

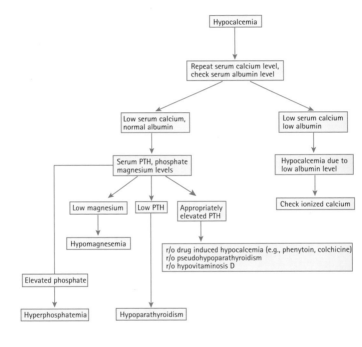

Diagnostic Imaging

Best Test(s)
• None

Ancillary Tests
• MRI of brain

Lab Evaluation

Best Test(s)
• LH, FSH
• Serum testosterone

Ancillary Tests
• Semen analysis
• Serum prolactin
• hCG stimulation
• Chromosome karyotype
• Seminal fluid fructose
• Testicular biopsy

Diagnostic Algorithm

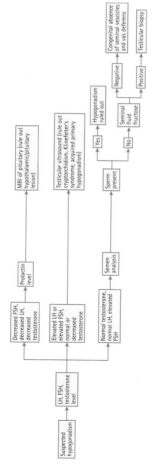

Diagnostic Imaging

Best Test(s)
• None

Ancillary Tests
• None

Lab Evaluation

Best Test(s)
• 24-hour urine potassium excretion

Ancillary Tests
• Serum electrolyte, BUN, creatinine
• Urine chloride
• Plasma renin, aldosterone

Diagnostic Algorithm

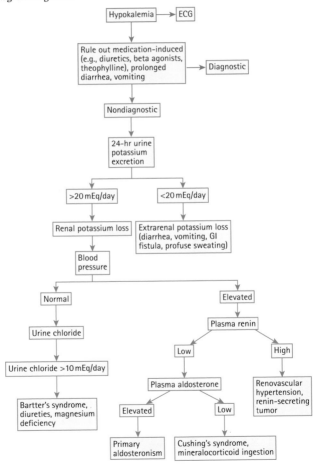

Diagnostic Imaging

Best Test(s)
• None

Ancillary Tests
• None

Lab Evaluation

Best Test(s)
• 24-hour urine magnesium level

Ancillary Tests
• Serum electrolytes, calcium, phosphate, glucose, albumin
• BUN, creatinine
• TSH
• Urine sodium

Diagnostic Algorithm

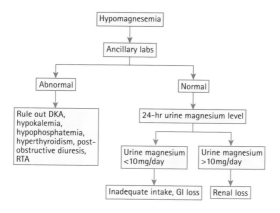

Diagnostic Imaging

Best Test(s)
• None

Ancillary Tests
• None

Lab Evaluation

Best Test(s)
• Serum electrolytes
• Serum osmolality

Ancillary Tests
• Serum glucose, BUN, creatinine
• Uric acid
• Urine osmolality
• TSH
• Serum cortisol
• Urinary sodium excretion

Diagnostic Algorithm

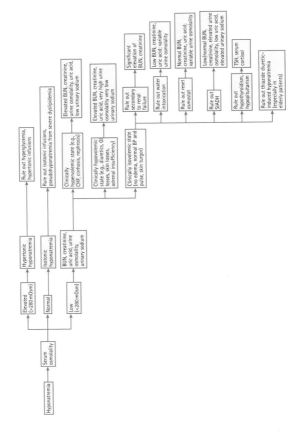

Diagnostic Imaging

Best Test(s)
• None

Ancillary Tests
• None

Lab Evaluation

Best Test(s)
• 24-hour urine phosphate excretion

Ancillary Tests
• Serum calcium, electrolytes, creatinine, glucose
• ABGs

Diagnostic Algorithm

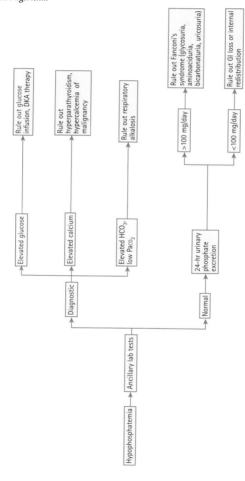

Diagnostic Imaging

Best Test(s)
• None

Ancillary Tests
• MRI of pituitary with contrast if secondary hypothyroidism is suspected

Lab Evaluation

Best Test(s)
• TSH

Ancillary Tests
• Antimicrosomal Ab if Hashimoto's thyroiditis is suspected
• Serum thyroglobulin level when subacute thyroiditis is suspected
• Free T_4

Diagnostic Algorithm

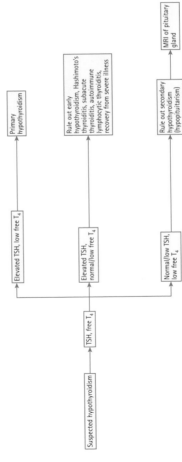

Diagnostic Imaging

Best Test(s)
• None

Ancillary Tests
• MRI of pituitary with contrast
• Hysterosalpingography
• Testicular ultrasound

Lab Evaluation

Best Test(s)
• Male: semen analysis
• Female: endometrial biopsy

Ancillary Tests
• FSH, LH
• Prolactin
• Serum testosterone (male)
• TSH
• CBC, ESR, FBS
• Urinalysis, VDRL, *Mycoplasma* culture, chlamydiae serology

Diagnostic Algorithm

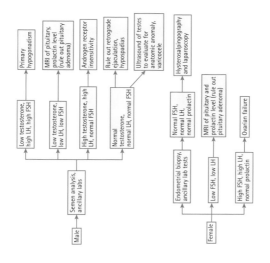

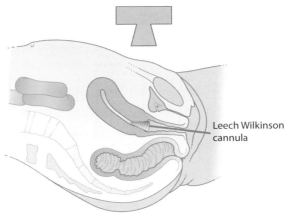

Leech Wilkinson cannula

A

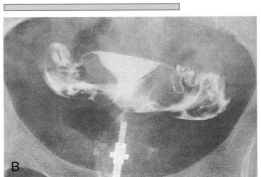

B

Figure 3-15 **A,** Hysterosalpingography enables assessment of the site of tubal obstruction and the presence of pathology in the uterine cavity. **B,** The triangular outline of the uterine cavity and the spill of dye on both sides from the fimbrial ends of the fallopian tubes can be seen. The dye spreads over the adjacent bowel. *(From Symonds EM, Symonds IM: Essential Obstetrics and Gynecology, ed 4, Edinburgh, Churchill Livingstone, 2004.)*

Diagnostic Imaging

Best Test(s)
• Abdominal CT or MRI with contrast

Ancillary Tests
• Octreotide scan

Lab Evaluation

Best Test(s)
• FBS
• Insulin level
• C peptide
• Plasma sulfonylurea assay

Ancillary Tests
• None

Diagnostic Algorithm

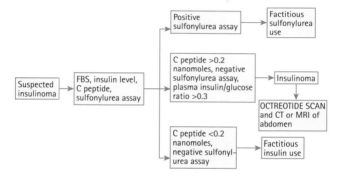

Diagnostic Imaging

Best Test(s)
• MRI of brain with IV contrast

Ancillary Tests
• CT of brain with contrast if MRI is
  contraindicated; CT of brain without
  contrast is not useful except for
  evaluation of bony erosions or
  calcifications

Lab Evaluation

Best Test(s)
• None

Ancillary Tests
• None

Diagnostic Algorithm

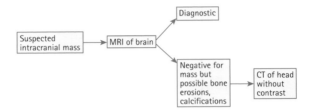

Diagnostic Imaging

Best Test(s)
- CT of abdomen with contrast if painless jaundice
- Ultrasound of abdomen if painful jaundice

Ancillary Tests
- ERCP
- MRCP
- Endoscopy ultrasound (EUS)

Lab Evaluation

Best Test(s)
- Bilirubin with fractionation
- Alkaline phosphatase, ALT, AST
- Viral hepatitis panel

Ancillary Tests
- Serum amylase, lipase, LDH
- CBC, reticulocyte count, Coombs' test
- BUN, creatinine, electrolytes
- Liver biopsy

Diagnostic Algorithm

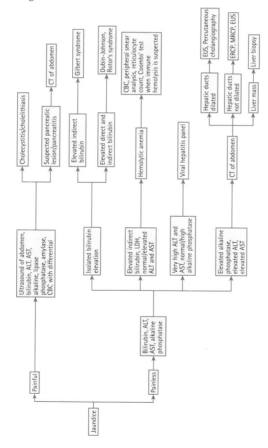

Diagnostic Imaging

Best Test(s)
• Radiograph of affected joint if history of trauma

Ancillary Tests
• MRI of affected joint if ligament tear is suspected
• CT if suspected fracture not visible on plain films

Lab Evaluation

Best Test(s)
• Arthrocentesis with fluid analysis (Gram stain, C&S, cell count and differential, examination for crystals under polarized light)

Ancillary Tests
• Lyme disease serology (western blot) in endemic areas
• Thayer-Martin culture
• Anaerobic cultures
• TB and fungal cultures

Diagnostic Algorithm

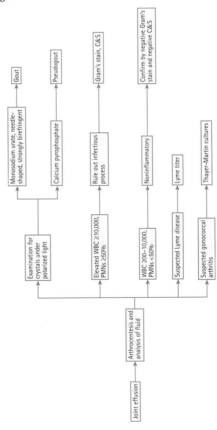

Diagnostic Imaging

Best Test(s)
• MRI of knee if history of trauma

Ancillary Tests
• Plain film of knee

Lab Evaluation

Best Test(s)
• Arthrocentesis and synovial fluid
  analysis of joint effusion

Ancillary Tests
• Uric acid
• ESR
• CBC with differential
• Lyme disease serology (western blot)

Diagnostic Algorithm

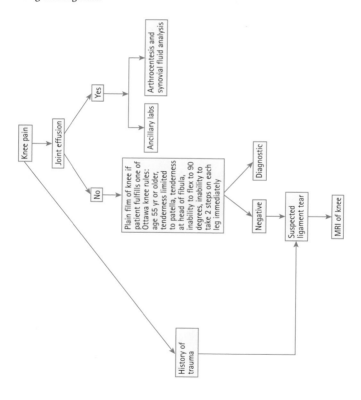

Diagnostic Imaging

Best Test(s)
- CT of liver with IV contrast

Ancillary Tests
- Ultrasound of liver if CT is contraindicated

Lab Evaluation

Best Test(s)
- Gram stain and C&S of abscess content is aspirated

Ancillary Tests
- ALT, AST (increased in 50% of cases)
- Alkaline phosphatase (increased in 95% of cases)
- Stool samples for *Entamoeba histolytica* trophozoites
- Serum antibody for *E. histolytica*

Diagnostic Algorithm

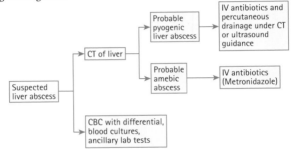

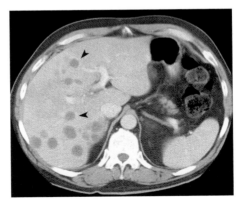

Figure 3-16 Liver abscess. Portal phase CT examination demonstrates multiple low-attenuation lesions with ring enhancement *(arrowheads).* The appearances are often non-specific on CT and often overlap with those of metastatic deposits. *(From Grainger RG, Allison DJ, Adam A, Dixon AK, eds: Grainger & Allison's Diagnostic Radiology, ed 4, Churchill Livingstone, Philadelphia, 2001.)*

Diagnostic Imaging

Best Test(s)
• Ultrasound of liver

Ancillary Tests
• CT of liver with contrast if ultrasound is inconclusive

Lab Evaluation

Best Test(s)
• Liver biopsy

Ancillary Tests
• ALT, AST, alkaline phosphatase
• Bilirubin
• GGTP
• Hepatitis panel
• Albumin level, PT
• ANA, transferrin saturation
• Serum protein IEP
• Ceruloplasmin level
• Serum copper, smooth muscle antibody, LKM-1 antibody

Diagnostic Algorithm

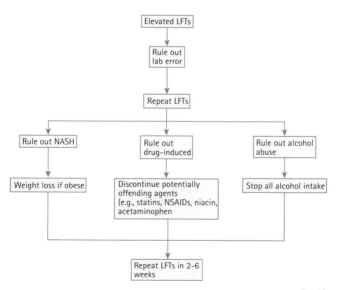

Cont'd

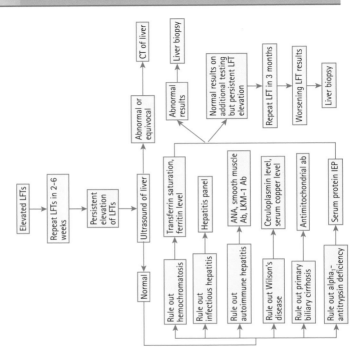

Diagnostic Imaging

Best Test(s)
• Ultrasound of liver

Ancillary Tests
• CT of liver
• MRI of liver

Lab Evaluation

Best Test(s)
• None

Ancillary Tests
• ALT, AST, alkaline phosphatase
• CBC with differential
• PT (INR)
• Hepatitis screen
• Alpha-fetoprotein level

Diagnostic Algorithm

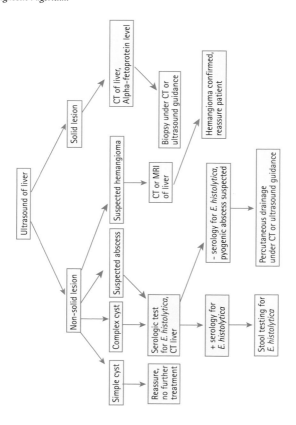

Diagnostic Imaging

Best Test(s)
- CT of chest with IV contrast

Ancillary Tests
- Chest radiograph may reveal cavitary lesion with air-fluid level

Lab Evaluation

Best Test(s)
- Gram stain and C&S of abscess material obtained at bronchoscopy

Ancillary Tests
- CBC with differential
- Blood culture × 2
- Sputum Gram stain and C&S (low yield)

Diagnostic Algorithm

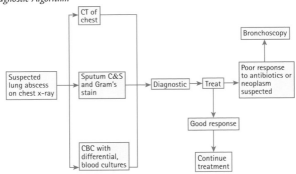

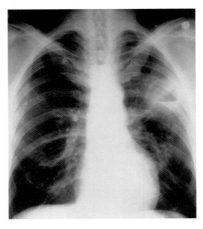

Figure 3-17 A lung abscess showing an air-fluid level. *(From Cohen J, Powderly WG: Infectious Diseases, ed 2, St. Louis, Mosby, 2004.)*

Diagnostic Imaging

Best Test(s)
• None

Ancillary Tests
• Mammogram (females)
• Chest radiograph or chest CT
• Ultrasound of axilla

Lab Evaluation

Best Test(s)
• Lymph node biopsy

Ancillary Tests
• CBC with differential
• HIV, monospot, viral titers
  (CMV, EB)

Diagnostic Algorithm

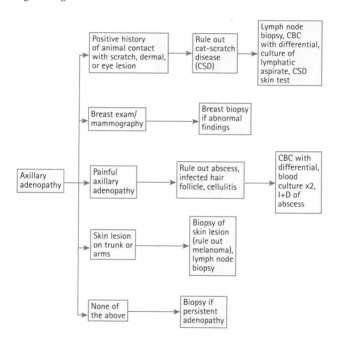

Diagnostic Imaging

Best Test(s)
• None

Ancillary Tests
• Chest radiograph
• CT of neck with IV contrast

Lab Evaluation

Best Test(s)
• Lymph node biopsy

Ancillary Tests
• CBC with differential
• Viral titers (EB, CMV)
• *Toxoplasma* titer
• Throat C&S

Diagnostic Algorithm

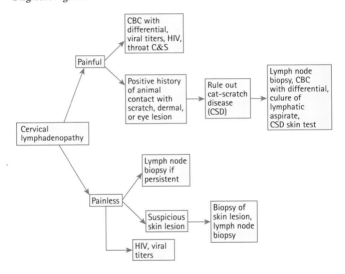

Diagnostic Imaging

Best Test(s)
• None

Ancillary Tests
• Chest radiograph

Lab Evaluation

Best Test(s)
• Lymph node biopsy

Ancillary Tests
• CBC with differential
• Biopsy of suspicious skin lesions on forearm, hand (r/o melanoma)
• VDRL, HIV

Diagnostic Algorithm

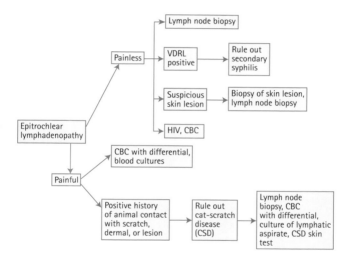

Diagnostic Imaging

Best Test(s)
• None

Ancillary Tests
• Chest radiograph
• CT of chest/abdomen/pelvis with IV contrast

Lab Evaluation

Best Test(s)
• Lymph node biopsy

Ancillary Tests
• CBC with differential
• HIV, viral titers (EB, CMV)
• *Toxoplasma* titers
• ALT, AST
• Blood culture × 2
• Bone marrow exam
• VDRL
• ESR (nonspecific)

Diagnostic Algorithm

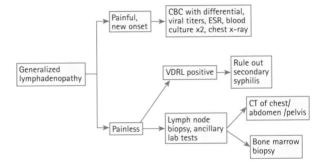

Diagnostic Imaging

Best Test(s)
• None

Ancillary Tests
• CT of abdomen/pelvis with IV contrast

Lab Evaluation

Best Test(s)
• Lymph node biopsy

Ancillary Tests
• CBC with differential
• VDRL
• Serology testing for *Chlamydia trachomatis*
• HIV
• ESR (nonspecific)
• Gonorrhea culture on Thayer-Martin medium
• HSV cultures
• Biopsy of skin lesions (r/o melanoma)

Diagnostic Algorithm

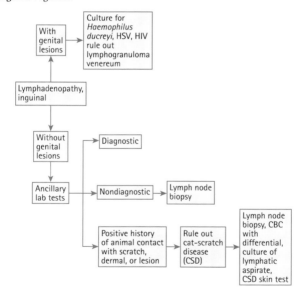

Diagnostic Imaging

Best Test(s)
- Lymphoscintigraphy (sensitivity and specificity of 100% in diagnosing lymphedema)

Ancillary Tests
- CT of abdomen/pelvis with IV contrast to exclude malignancy leading to obstruction
- Lymphangiography (rarely used and difficult to perform; may be requested by surgeon considering repair or excision of tissue for lymphedema)

Lab Evaluation

Best Test(s)
- None

Ancillary Tests
- BUN, creatinine, ALT, AST
- Serum albumin
- TSH

Diagnostic Algorithm

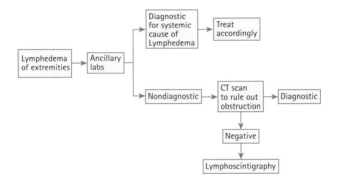

Diagnostic Imaging

Best Test(s)
• None

Ancillary Tests
• None

Lab Evaluation

Best Test(s)
• Reticulocyte count

Ancillary Tests
• Serum B$_{12}$ level
• Serum folate level
• TSH
• ALT, AST
• LDH, bilirubin, serum haptoglobin,
• ANA, Coomb's test if suspected
  hemolytic anemia

Diagnostic Algorithm

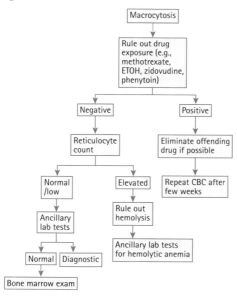

Diagnostic Imaging

Best Test(s)
• Small-bowel series

Ancillary Tests
• CT of pancreas with IV contrast
• Video capsule endoscopy

Lab Evaluation

Best Test(s)
• Biopsy of small bowel

Ancillary Tests
• Albumin, total protein
• ALT, AST, PT (INR)
• Serum electrolytes, BUN, creatinine
• Sudan III stain of stool for fecal leukocytes
• CBC, RBC folate, serum iron, serum carotene, cholesterol, serum calcium
• Hydrogen 14-C xylose breath test
• D-Xylose test, secretin test
• Quantitative fecal test
• Antigliadin antibody, IgA endomysial antibody

Diagnostic Algorithm

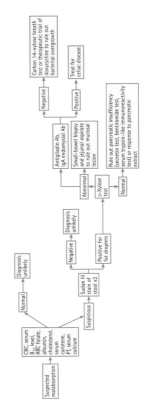

Diagnostic Imaging

Best Test(s)
- CT of mastoid process with contrast (can demonstrate mastoiditis with bone destruction)

Ancillary Tests
- Plain radiograph of mastoid region (may demonstrate clouding or opacification)
- MRI with contrast (more sensitive than CT scan in evaluating soft tissue involvement and useful in conjunction with CT scan to investigate other complications of mastoiditis)

Lab Evaluation

Best Test(s)
- Gram stain and C&S of fluid obtained by myringotomy or drainage from tympanic membrane

Ancillary Tests
- CBC with differential

Diagnostic Algorithm

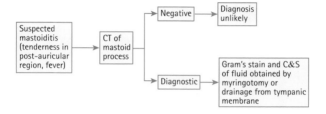

Diagnostic Imaging

Best Test(s)
• Tc-99m radionuclide scan (Meckel scan)

Ancillary Tests
• Ultrasound or CT of abdomen/pelvis

Lab Evaluation

Best Test(s)
• None

Ancillary Tests
• CBC with differential

Diagnostic Algorithm

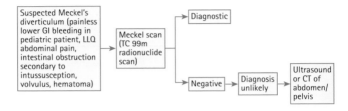

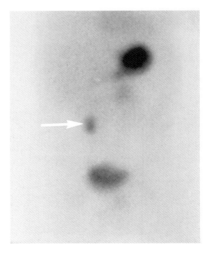

Figure 3-18 Radionuclide image of Meckel's diverticulum. Increased radionuclide uptake by ectopic gastric mucosa *(arrow)* in the Meckel's diverticulum. The patient was an 11-month-old boy who presented with acute bleeding. (Courtesy of Dr. Kieran McHugh and reproduced with permission from Nolan DJ: *Schweiz Med Wochenschr* 128:109-114, 1998.) *(From Grainger RG, Allison DJ, Adam A, Dixon AK, eds: Grainger & Allison's Diagnostic Radiology, ed 4, Philadelphia, 2001, Churchill Livingstone.)*

Diagnostic Imaging

Best Test(s)
• CT of chest with IV contrast

Ancillary Tests
• None

Lab Evaluation

Best Test(s)
• Lymph node biopsy

Ancillary Tests
• CBC
• ESR (nonspecific)
• ALT, AST
• PPD
• Serum ACE level

Diagnostic Algorithm

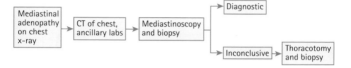

Mediastinal adenopathy on chest x-ray → CT of chest, ancillary labs → Mediastinoscopy and biopsy → Diagnostic / Inconclusive → Thoracotomy and biopsy

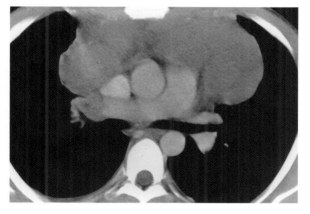

Figure 3-19 Mediastinal masses in lymphoma. Contrast-enhanced CT showing a large anterior mass in a young patient with Hodgkin's disease. No other disease was demonstrated. *(From Grainger RG, Allison DJ, Adam A, Dixon AK, eds: Grainger & Allison's Diagnostic Radiology, ed 4, Churchill Livingstone, Philadelphia, 2001.)*

Diagnostic Imaging

Best Test(s)
• MRI or CT of brain with contrast

Ancillary Tests
• Cerebral angiography

Lab Evaluation

Best Test(s)
• None

Ancillary Tests
• None

Diagnostic Algorithm

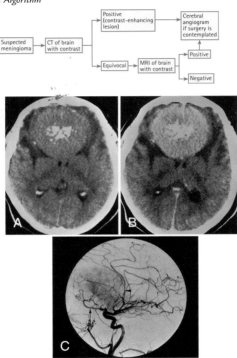

Figure 3-20 Subfrontal meningioma. CT before (**A**) and after (**B**) IV contrast medium, and lateral projection of common carotid anteriogram (**C**). There is a large circumscribed mass in the anterior cranial fossa that is isodense to normal gray matter, contains foci of calcification centrally, and enhances homogenously. There is edema in the white matter of both frontal lobes and posterior displacement and splaying of the frontal horns of the lateral ventricles. On the arteriogram (**C**) the mass is delineated by a tumor blush and there is posterior displacement of the anterior cerebral arteries *(arrowhead)*, mirroring the mass effect seen on CT. The ophthalmic artery is enlarged as its ethmoidal branches supply the tumor *(arrow)*. (*From Grainger RG, Allison DJ, Adam A, Dixon AK, eds: Grainger & Allison's Diagnostic Radiology, ed 4, Churchill Livingstone, Philadelphia, 2001.*)

Diagnostic Imaging

Best Test(s)
• None

Ancillary Tests
• CT of brain with contrast if focal neurologic deficts present on examination, patient is in coma, or papillary abnormalities or papilledema is noted
• MRI with contrast if sequelae are suspected (e.g., abscess)

Lab Evaluation

Best Test(s)
• LP and CSF examination (measure opening pressure, Gram stain, CSF protein, glucose, WBC with differential, and bacterial antigen)

Ancillary Tests
• CBC with differential
• Blood culture × 2

Diagnostic Algorithm

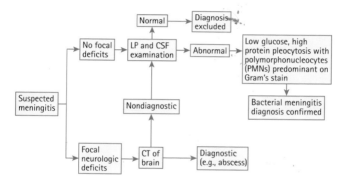

Diagnostic Imaging

Best Test(s)
- CT of abdomen with IV contrast (may reveal bowel wall thickening, venous dilation, venous thrombus)

Ancillary Tests
- Angiography if CT is inconclusive
- Abdominal plain radiograph (generally nonspecific)

Lab Evaluation

Best Test(s)
- CBC with differential
- Serum electrolytes (metabolic acidosis is indicative of possible bowel infarction)

Ancillary Tests
- Serum amylase
- Hypercoagulopathy workup (e.g., PT, PTT, platelets, protein C, protein S, antithrombin III)

Diagnostic Algorithm

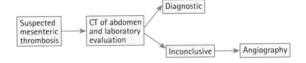

Diagnostic Imaging

Best Test(s)
• CT of chest with IV contrast

Ancillary Tests
• CT of abdomen with IV contrast and bone scan to assess extent of disease

Lab Evaluation

Best Test(s)
• Pleural biopsy

Ancillary Tests
• Cytology from diagnostic thoracentesis is generally inadequate for diagnosis
• PFTs

Diagnostic Algorithm

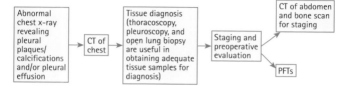

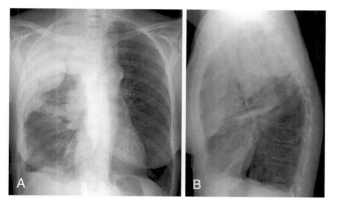

Figure 3-21 Malignant pleural thickening. PA **(A)** and lateral **(B)** chest radiographs. Malignant pleural thickening is characteristically lobulated and nodular. The extensive right-sided disease in this patient was caused by mesothelioma. Notice the extension of the tumor into the fissure *(arrows)*. *(From Grainger RG, Allison DJ, Adam A, Dixon AK, eds: Grainger & Allison's Diagnostic Radiology, ed 4, Churchill Livingstone, Philadelphia, 2001.)*

Diagnostic Imaging

Best Test(s)
• None

Ancillary Tests
• Chest radiograph

Lab Evaluation

Best Test(s)
• Serum electrolytes
• ABGs

Ancillary Tests
• BUN, creatinine, glucose
• Determination of anion gapAG =
  $Na^+ - (Cl^- + HCO_3)$

Diagnostic Algorithm

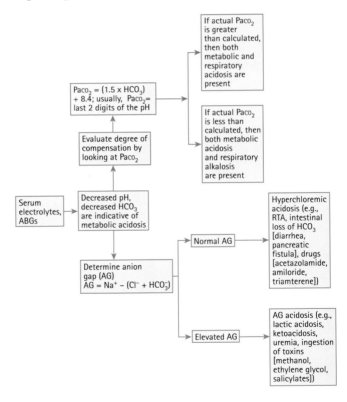

Diagnostic Imaging

Best Test(s)
• None

Ancillary Tests
• Chest radiograph

Lab Evaluation

Best Test(s)
• Serum electrolytes
• ABGs

Ancillary Tests
• BUN, creatinine
• Urine chloride level

Diagnostic Algorithm

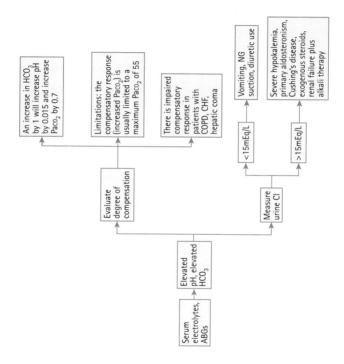

Diagnostic Imaging

Best Test(s)
• None

Ancillary Tests
• None

Lab Evaluation

Best Test(s)
• Red blood cell distribution width (RDW)

Ancillary Tests
• Reticulocyte count
• Ferritin level,
• TIBC, serum iron
• Hemoglobin electrophoresis

Diagnostic Algorithm

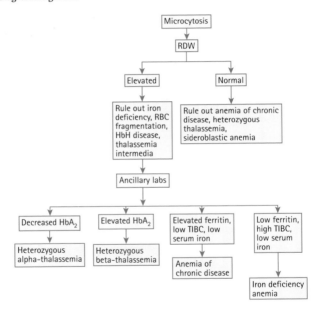

Diagnostic Imaging

Best Test(s)
• None

Ancillary Tests
• Plain radiographs of painful areas may demonstrate punched-out lytic lesions
• Bone scan is not useful because lesions are not blastic
• Ultrasound of kidneys if renal insufficiency present

Lab Evaluation

Best Test(s)
• Serum and urine protein IEP
• Bone marrow exam

Ancillary Tests
• CBC and peripheral smear (normochromic, normocytic anemia, rouleaux formation, thrombocytopenia)
• Serum calcium (elevated)
• Urinalysis (proteinuria)
• BUN, creatinine, uric acid, LDH, total protein (all elevated)
• Serum electrolytes (decreased anion gap, hyponatremia)

Diagnostic Algorithm

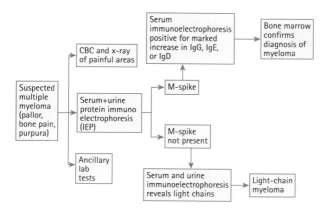

Diagnostic Imaging

Best Test(s)
• MRI of brain with gadolinium

Ancillary Tests
• MRI of C-spine with gadolinium in selected cases

Lab Evaluation

Best Test(s)
• LP with CSF analysis

Ancillary Tests
• Agarose electrophoresis of CSF (reveals discrete "oligoclonal" bands in the gamma region in approximately 90% of cases)
• Elevated CSF protein, mononuclear WBC, gamma globulin (mostly IgG)
• Presence of myelin basic protein in CSF

Diagnostic Algorithm

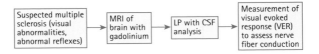

T2W   Gd T1W

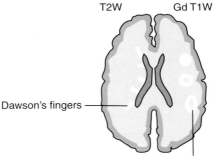

Dawson's fingers

Enhancing plaques

Figure 3-22 Multiple sclerosis MRI findings. *(From Weissleder R, Wittenberg J, Harisinghani MG, Chen JW: Primer of Diagnostic Imaging, ed 4, St. Louis, Mosby, 2007.)*

Diagnostic Imaging

Best Test(s)
• None

Ancillary Tests
• None

Lab Evaluation

Best Test(s)
• CPK (with fractionation if elevated)

Ancillary Tests
• Serum aldolase
• Serum electrolytes, BUN, creatinine, calcium, magnesium, phosphate, glucose
• TSH, ANA, ESR
• Muscle biopsy

Diagnostic Algorithm

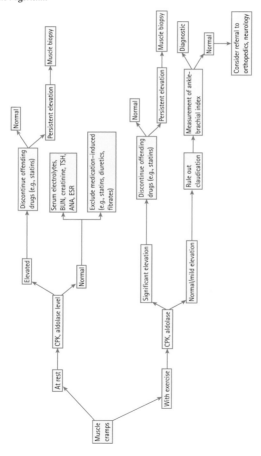

Diagnostic Imaging

Best Test(s)
• None

Ancillary Tests
• None

Lab Evaluation

Best Test(s)
• Muscle biopsy

Ancillary Tests
• CBC with differential
• CPK, aldolase
• ESR (nonspecific)
• TSH
• Serum electrolytes, BUN, creatinine, glucose, calcium
• B_{12} level, ANA

Diagnostic Algorithm

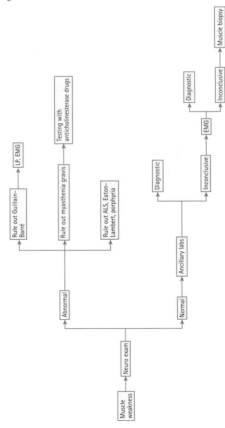

Diagnostic Imaging

Best Test(s)
• None

Ancillary Tests
• CT scan of chest with IV contrast to r/o thymoma (found in 12% of patients with MG)

Lab Evaluation

Best Test(s)
• AChR-Ab (present in 90% of patients with generalized MG and 60% of patients with ocular MG); indicated only if testing with anticholinesterase medications supports diagnosis of MG

Ancillary Tests
• TSH, free T_4 (to r/o thyroid disease, which occurs in 5% to 15% of patients with MG)
• B_{12} level
• ANA, rheumatoid factor (increased association of MG with SLE, rheumatoid arthritis)

Diagnostic Algorithm

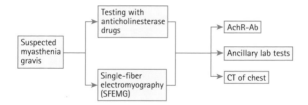

Diagnostic Imaging

Best Test(s)
• Radionuclide stress test

Ancillary Tests
• Stress echocardiogram
• Chest radiograph
• ECG
• Cardiac catheterization

Lab Evaluation

Best Test(s)
• Cardiac troponins
• CPK-MB × 2

Ancillary Tests
• Lipid panel
• Glucose, creatinine
• CBC

Diagnostic Algorithm

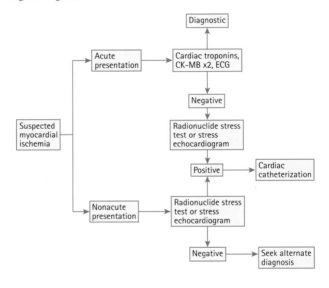

Diagnostic Imaging

Best Test(s)
• CT or MRI of neck

Ancillary Tests
• Thyroid ultrasound
• Chest radiograph

Lab Evaluation

Best Test(s)
• None

Ancillary Tests
• CBC with differential
• TSH
• Serum calcium
• Monospot
• Throat C&S

Diagnostic Algorithm

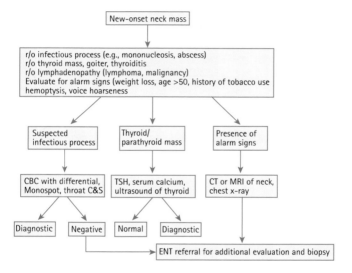

Diagnostic Imaging

Best Test(s)
- None

Ancillary Tests
- CT of abdomen with IV contrast

Lab Evaluation

Best Test(s)
- Bone marrow exam

Ancillary Tests
- CBC with differential
- HIV
- Blood culture × 2, urine C&S
- B_{12} level, folate

Diagnostic Algorithm

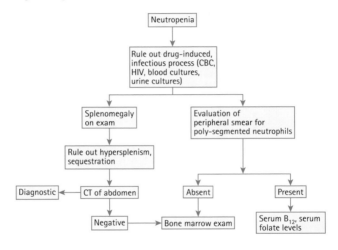

Diagnostic Imaging

Best Test(s)
• Ultrasound of kidneys and urinary bladder
• Urinalysis

Ancillary Tests
• Spiral CT of abdomen/pelvis

Lab Evaluation

Best Test(s)
• Urinalysis

Ancillary Tests
• BUN, creatinine, serum electrolytes
• Serum osmolality
• Urine osmolality, urine sodium
• 24-hour urine collection for protein
• CBC

Diagnostic Algorithm

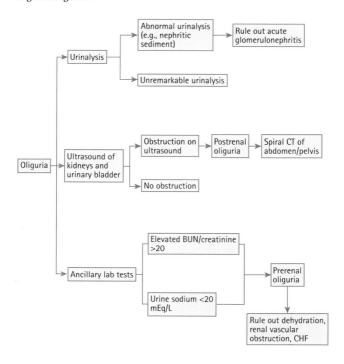

Diagnostic Imaging

Best Test(s)
• MRI of affected bone with contrast

Ancillary Tests
• Three-phase bone scan with Tc 99m MDP (useful if MRI is contraindicated or is not readily available)
• Doppler study of affected extremity (useful for determining vascular patency in selected patients [e.g., diabetics])
• Conventional radiograph of affected bone (initial imaging test)

Lab Evaluation

Best Test(s)
• Bone culture following surgical débridement

Ancillary Tests
• ESR
• CBC with differential
• Blood culture 3 2

Diagnostic Algorithm

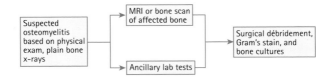

Figure

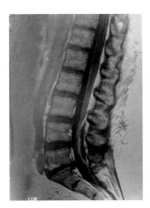

Figure 3-23 Vertebral osteomyelitis. A sagittal, contrast-enhanced conventional spin echo MRI scan (T1-weighted) demonstrates a posteriorly located epidural abscess at the L4-L5 vertebral level with an enhancing rim and displacement of the nerve roots anteriorly. *(Courtesy of Dr. Joseph Mammone. From Cohen J, Powderly WG: Infectious Diseases, ed 2, St. Louis, Mosby, 2004.)*

Diagnostic Imaging

Best Test(s)
- MRI of affected bone

Ancillary Tests
- CT scan of involved bone if MRI is contraindicated
- Bone scan (decreased uptake)

Lab Evaluation

Best Test(s)
- None

Ancillary Tests
- CBC
- ESR, ANA
- ALT, AST, creatinine

Diagnostic Algorithm

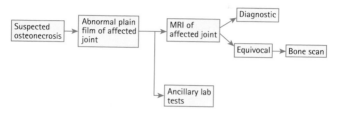

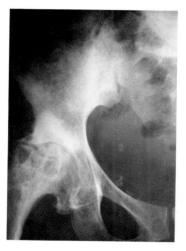

Figure 3-24 Advanced osteonecrosis of the femoral of the femoral head (Steinberg stages 5-6). Gross destruction and remodeling of the femoral head. There are significant osteoarthritic changes. *(From Hochberg MC, Silma AJ, Smolen JS, Weinblatt ME, Weisman MH, eds: Rheumatology, 3 ed, St. Louis, Mosby, 2003.)*

Diagnostic Imaging

Best Test(s)
- DEXA scan

Ancillary Tests
- Single-photon absorptiometry, dual-photon absorptiometry, or quantitative CT scan (DEXA scan is preferred)

Lab Evaluation

Best Test(s)
- None

Ancillary Tests
- TSH
- PTH, serum calcium, phosphate in selected cases
- Serum vitamin D 1,25 (OH)2D level

Diagnostic Algorithm

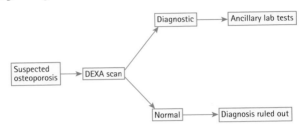

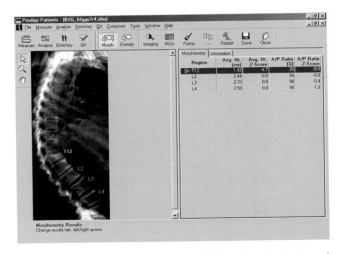

Figure 3-25. Vertebral fracture assessment from a dual x-ray absorptiometry image of the spine. Use of dual-energy images facilitates the visualization of the lumbar and thoracic spine in a single image. In this example, a fracture has been identified at T12. *(From Hochberg MC, Silma AJ, Smolen JS, Weinblatt ME, Weisman MH, eds: Rheumatology, 3 ed, St. Louis, Mosby, 2003.)*

Diagnostic Imaging

Best Test(s)
• Plain radiographs of affected bones (will show opacity and radiolucency)

Ancillary Tests
• Bone scan (will reveal activity and extent of disease)

Lab Evaluation

Best Test(s)
• Serum alkaline phosphatase (elevated)

Ancillary Tests
• Serum calcium, phosphate

Diagnostic Algorithm

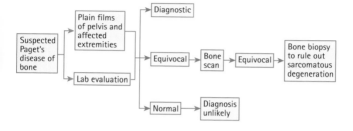

Diagnostic Imaging

Best Test(s)
• High-resolution CT of pancreas with IV contrast

Ancillary Tests
• MRI of abdomen if CT is equivocal
• Endoscopic ultrasound (EUS)
• ERCP

Lab Evaluation

Best Test(s)
• Tissue diagnosis

Ancillary Tests
• Alkaline phosphatase
• ALT, AST

Diagnostic Algorithm

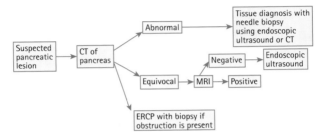

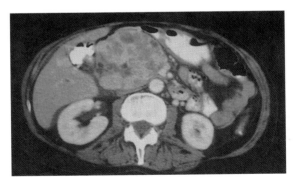

Figure 3-26 Pancreatic carcinoma on CT. *(From Talley NJ, Martin CJ: Clinical Gastroenterology, ed 2, Sidney, Churchill Livingstone, 2006.)*

Diagnostic Imaging

Best Test(s)
- High-resolution CT of pancreas with IV contrast

Ancillary Tests
- ERCP
- Endoscopic ultrasound (EUS)

Lab Evaluation

Best Test(s)
- Ultrasound-guided needle biopsy

Ancillary Tests
- Serum amylase, lipase
- Alkaline phosphatase, ALT
- Serum calcium

Diagnostic Algorithm

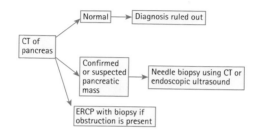

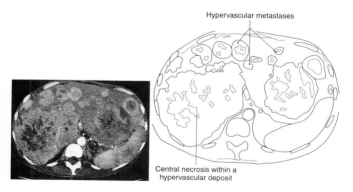

Figure 3-27 Liver metastases from a primary pancreatic carcinoid tumor: CT appearances. **A,** the CT scan performed at 25s following IV injection of contrast medium ("arterial" phase) shows typical hypervascular carcinoid liver metastases. The larger lesion in the right lobe shows central necrosis.

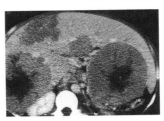

Primary tumor in the tail
of the pancreas

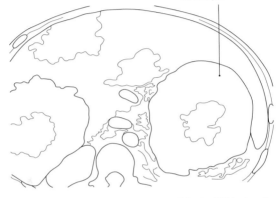

Figure 3-27 **B,** The CT scan performed at 75s following IV injection of
contrast medium ("portal venous" phase) shows that the vascular lesions
have now become isodense with the normal liver parenchyma. The primary tumor in the tail of the pancreas is also clearly seen. As depicted
here, carcinoid hepatic metastases are typically hypervascular and are
optimally depicted during the arterial phase of a contrast-enhanced CT
or MR scan as they are isoattenuating when compared with adjacent
hepatic parenchyma during the portal venous phase of enhancement.
*(From Besser CM, Thorner MO: Comprehensive Clinical Endocrinology,
ed 3, St. Louis, Mosby, 2002.)*

Diagnostic Imaging

Best Test(s)
- CT of abdomen with IV contrast

Ancillary Tests
- Ultrasound of abdomen when gallstone pancreatitis is suspected
- Abdominal plain film (often performed as initial imaging test in acute setting)
- Chest radiograph

Lab Evaluation

Best Test(s)
- Serum amylase
- Serum lipase

Ancillary Tests
- Serum trypsin level and urinary trypsinogen level (sensitive tests but not readily available)
- ALT, AST, serum calcium, glucose, electrolytes, alkaline phosphatase but not readily
- CBC, urinalysis
- ABGs

Diagnostic Algorithm

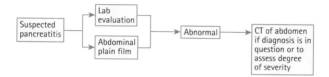

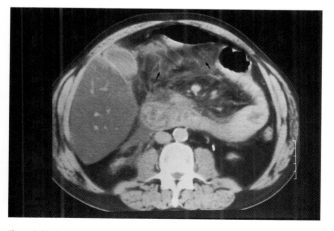

Figure 3-28 Spread of acute pancreatitis. Enhanced CT demonstrates the inflammatory changes of acute pancreatitis spreading along the transverse mesocolon *(arrows)* toward the transverse colon. Phlegmonous extension through the small-bowel mesentery is also present. *(From Grainger RG, Allison DJ, Adam A, Dixon AK, eds: Grainger & Allison's Diagnostic Radiology, ed 4, Churchill Livingstone, Philadelphia, 2001.)*

Diagnostic Imaging

Best Test(s)
• CT of pelvis with IV contrast

Ancillary Tests
• Ultrasound of pelvis if CT is
  contraindicated

Lab Evaluation

Best Test(s)
• Gram stain and C&S of abscess

Ancillary Tests
• CBC with differential
• Aerobic and anaerobic cultures of
  cervix, blood, peritoneal cavity
  (if entered)
• Urinalysis, urine C&S
• Pregnancy test in reproductive age
  female

Diagnostic Algorithm

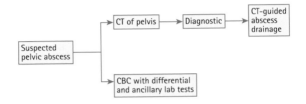

Diagnostic Imaging

Best Test(s)
• Ultrasound of pelvis is best initial study

Ancillary Tests
• CT of pelvis with IV contrast
• MRI of pelvis

Lab Evaluation

Best Test(s)
• Biopsy of pelvic mass

Ancillary Tests
• CA 125
• CBC, creatinine
• Serum hCG

Diagnostic Algorithm

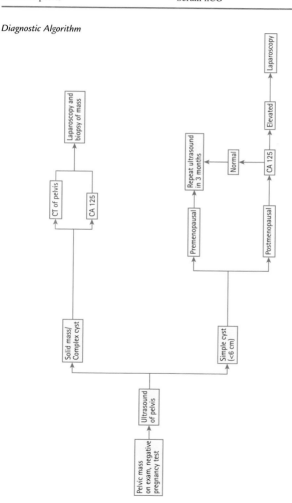

Diagnostic Imaging

Best Test(s)
• Ultrasound of pelvis

Ancillary Tests
• Spiral CT of abdomen/pelvis with IV contrast

Lab Evaluation

Best Test(s)
• Serum hCG

Ancillary Tests
• Urinalysis, urine C&S
• CBC with differential
• GC serology cultures, blood culture × 2

Diagnostic Algorithm

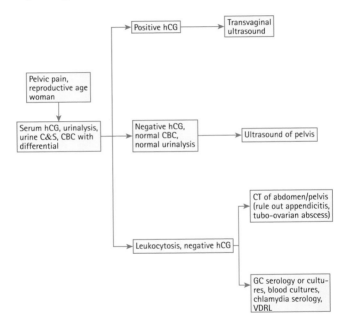

Diagnostic Imaging

Best Test(s)
• None

Ancillary Tests
• UGI series if patient refuses endoscopy
• Abdominal ultrasound in suspected cholelithiasis/cholecystitis
• CT of abdomen if suspected pancreatic lesion

Lab Evaluation

Best Test(s)
• None

Ancillary Tests
• *H. pylori* stool antigen test or urea breath test
• CBC
• Serum amylase if acute abdominal pain

Diagnostic Algorithm

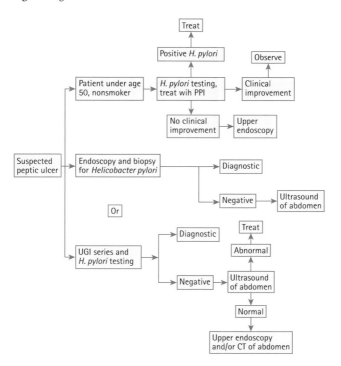

Diagnostic Imaging

Best Test(s)
- Continuous wave Doppler to measure systolic arterial pressure and Ankle Brachial Index (ABI)

Ancillary Tests
- Doppler ultrasound (can be used to locate occluded areas and assess patency of distal arterial system
- Angiography (if surgical reconstruction is being considered, for angioplasty, or for stent placement)

Lab Evaluation

Best Test(s)
- None

Ancillary Tests
- FBS
- Lipid panel
- Creatinine

Diagnostic Algorithm

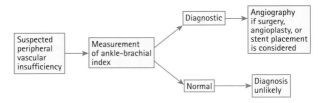

Diagnostic Imaging

Best Test(s)
• None

Ancillary Tests
• Chest radiograph (useful to r/o sarcoidosis, lung carcinoma)
• Plain bone films in suspected trauma

Lab Evaluation

Best Test(s)
• None

Ancillary Tests
• CBC, glucose, electrolytes, ALT, AST, calcium, magnesium, phosphate
• Heavy metal screening in suspected toxic neuropathy
• Lyme Disease Serology in endemic areas or in patients with suggestive history and physical exam erythema chronicum migrans (ECM)
• TSH, B_{12}, folate level
• HIV in patients with risk factors

Diagnostic Algorithm

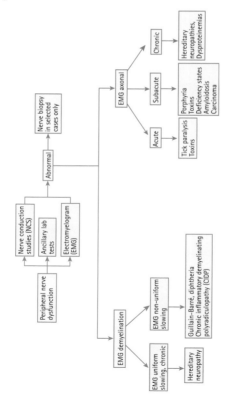

Diagnostic Imaging

Best Test(s)
• None; imaging generally not indicated unless abscess is extensive

Ancillary Tests
• CT of pelvis with IV contrast
• Endoscopy ultrasound (EUS)

Lab Evaluation

Best Test(s)
• Gram stain, C&S of abscess (aerobic and anaerobic cultures)

Ancillary Tests
• CBC with differential
• Blood culture × 2

Diagnostic Algorithm

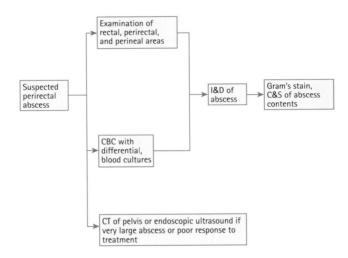

Diagnostic Imaging

Best Test(s)
- Scintigraphy with iodine-131-I MIBG (100% sensitivity); this norepinephrine analogue localizes in adrenergic tissue and is particularly useful in locating extra-adrenal pheochromocytomas

Ancillary Tests
- MRI of abdomen with IV contrast
- 6[18F]-fluorodopamine PET (reserved for cases in which clinical symptoms and signs suggest pheochromocytoma and results of biochemical tests are positive, but conventional imaging studies cannot locate tumor)

Lab Evaluation

Best Test(s)
- Plasma free metanephrines (plasma concentration of normetanephrines > 2.5 pmol/ml or metanephrines > 1.4 pmol/ml indicate pheochromocytoma with 100% specificity)

Ancillary Tests
- 24-hour urine collection for metanephrines (elevated)
- Clonidine suppression test

Diagnostic Algorithm

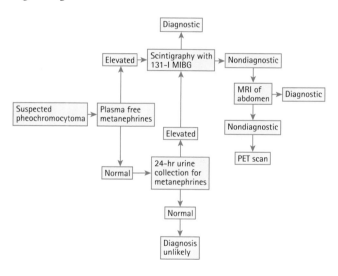

Diagnostic Imaging

Best Test(s)
• MRI of pituitary with gadolinium

Ancillary Tests
• CT of pituitary if MRI is contraindicated

Lab Evaluation

Best Test(s)
• Tests for hormonal excess or deficit based on clinical presentation (e.g., serum prolactin level, IGF-I, free T$_4$, dexamethasone suppression test)

Ancillary Tests
• None

Diagnostic Algorithm

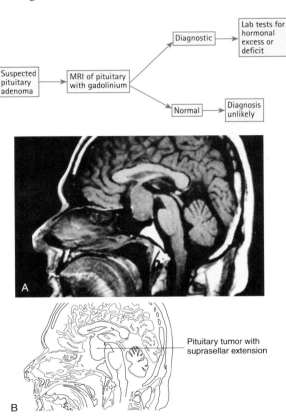

Figure 3-29 MRI showing a large pituitary tumor with suprasellar extension causing acromegaly. (*From Besser CM, Thorner MO: Comprehensive Clinical Endocrinology, ed 3, St. Louis, Mosby, 2002.*)

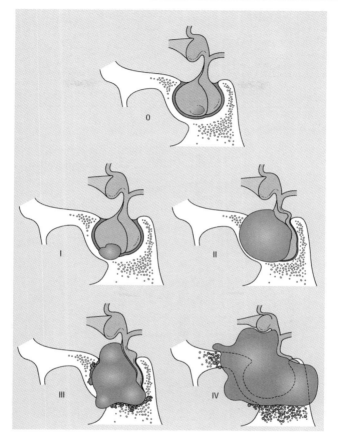

Figure 3-30 Radiologic classification of pituitary adenomas. Pituitary tumors are commonly classified on the basis of their size, invasion status, and growth patterns, as proposed by Hardy and Vezina in 1979. Tumors less than or equal to 1 cm in diameter are designated microadenomas, whereas larger tumors are designated macroadenomas. Grade 0: Intrapituitary microadenoma; normal sellar appearance. Grade 1: Intrapituitary microadenoma; focal bulging of sellar wall. Grade 2: Intrasellar macroadenoma; diffusely enlarged sella; no invasion. Grade 3: Macroadenoma; localized sellar invasion and/or destruction. Grade 4: Macroadenoma; extensive sellar invasion and/or destruction. Tumors are further subclassified on the basis of their extrasellar extension, whether suprasellar or parasellar. *(From Besser CM, Thorner MO: Comprehensive Clinical Endocrinology, ed 3, St. Louis, Mosby, 2002.)*

Diagnostic Imaging

Best Test(s)
• Obstetric ultrasound

Ancillary Tests
• MRI (has been effective in detecting placenta previa; however, sonography remains preferred method of diagnosis)

Lab Evaluation

Best Test(s)
• None

Ancillary Tests
• CBC

Diagnostic Algorithm

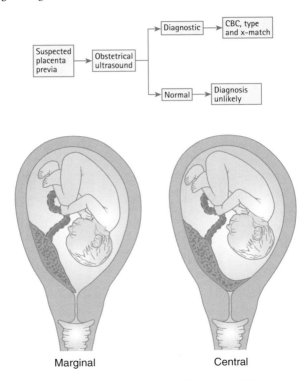

Figure 3-31 Classification of placenta previa. (*From Symonds EM, Symonds IM: Essential Obstetrics and Gynecology, ed 4, Edinburgh, Churchill Livingstone, 2004.*)

Diagnostic Imaging

Best Test(s)
• Chest radiograph

Ancillary Tests
• CT of chest without contrast
• Ultrasound (if necessary) for diagnostic thoracentesis

Lab Evaluation

Best Test(s)
• Diagnostic thoracentesis and pleural fluid analysis for pH, LDH, glucose, cell count, protein

Ancillary Tests
• Serum total protein, albumin, LDH, glucose
• CBC
• Pleural biopsy
• Adenosine deaminase (ADA)
• Cytologic analysis

Diagnostic Algorithm

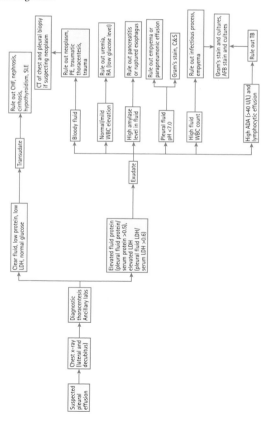

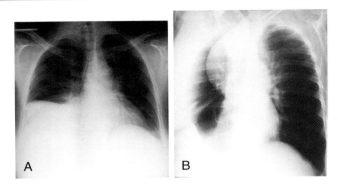

Figure 3-32 Subpulmonary pleural effusion. **A,** On the erect PA film the effusion simulates a high hemidiaphragm. **B,** A right lateral decubitus view demonstrates the fluid *(arrows)*. *(From Grainger RG, Allison DJ, Adam A, Dixon AK, eds: Grainger & Allison's Diagnostic Radiology, ed 4, Churchill Livingstone, Philadelphia, 2001.)*

Diagnostic Imaging

Best Test(s)
- Abdominal arteriogram (reveals small or large aneurysms and arteries focal constrictions between dilated segments, usually in renal, mesenteric, or hepatic arteries)

Ancillary Tests
- CT or ultrasound of abdomen to exclude other causes

Lab Evaluation

Best Test(s)
- Biopsy of small or medium-sized artery (biopsies of gastrocnemius muscle and sural nerve are commonly performed)

Ancillary Tests
- ESR, CBC
- HBsAg, ANA
- ALT, BUN, creatinine
- pANCA

Diagnostic Algorithm

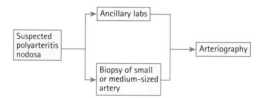

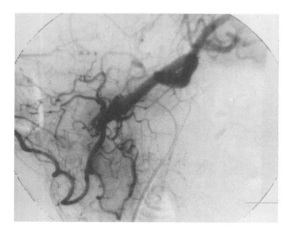

Figure 3-33 Aneurysms on the mesenteric artery in polyarteritis. *(From Hochberg MC, Silma AJ, Smolen JS, Weinblatt ME, Weisman MH, eds: Rheumatology, ed 3, St. Louis, Mosby, 2003.)*

Diagnostic Imaging

Best Test(s)
• Renal ultrasound

Ancillary Tests
• CT or MRI of kidneys (more sensitive than ultrasound and indicated if there are concerns regarding solid lesions)

Lab Evaluation

Best Test(s)
• None

Ancillary Tests
• CBC (erythrocytosis secondary to elevated erythropoietin level)
• BUN, creatinine, electrolytes, urinalysis
• Serum erythropoietin level
• Genetic testing: defective *PKD1* gene locus—chromosome 16 or chromosome 4 (*PKD2*)

Diagnostic Algorithm

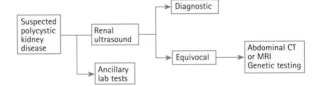

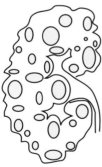

Polycystic kidney

Figure 3-34 Polycystic kidney disease. (*From Weissleder R, Wittenberg J, Harisinghani MG, Chen JW: Primer of Diagnostic Imaging, ed 4, St. Louis, Mosby, 2007.*)

Diagnostic Imaging

Best Test(s)
• None

Ancillary Tests
• CT of abdomen with IV contrast to r/o carcinoma of kidney and liver and polycystic kidney disease and to evaluate for splenomegaly
• RBC mass measurement if stress polycythemia is suspected

Lab Evaluation

Best Test(s)
• Serum erythropoietin level (low)
• Peripheral blood JAK2 V617 mutation screen

Ancillary Tests
• Leukocyte alkaline phosphatase (increased), B_{12} level (increased), uric acid level (increased)
• O_2 saturation
• P50, blood (oxygen dissociation curve)

Diagnostic Algorithm

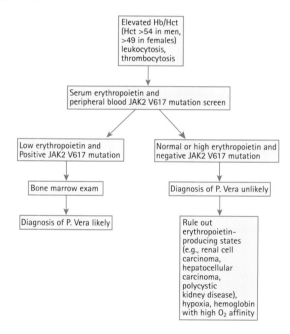

Diagnostic Imaging

Best Test(s)
• Duplex Doppler ultrasound of abdomen

Ancillary Tests
• CT or MRI of abdomen can be done when sonogram results are equivocal
• MRA (useful for detection of portal vein obstruction)
• Upper endoscopy (r/o esophageal/gastric varices)

Lab Evaluation

Best Test(s)
• None

Ancillary Tests
• CBC, platelet count
• Viral hepatitis screen
• ALT, AST, PT, PTT, albumin
• Anti-smooth muscle Ab, antimitochondrial Ab, ceruloplasmin level, serum protein IEP

Diagnostic Algorithm

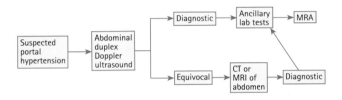

Diagnostic Imaging

Best Test(s)
• Doppler ultrasound of portal vein

Ancillary Tests
• MRI of portal vein if Doppler ultrasound is equivocal
• Abdominal CT with IV contrast (r/o neoplasm)

Lab Evaluation

Best Test(s)
• None

Ancillary Tests
• CBC with differential
• Coagulopathy screen (PT, PTT, factor V leiden protein C, protein S, anti-thrombin III, lupus anticoagulant)
• ALT, AST, creatinine, urinalysis
• ANA

Diagnostic Algorithm

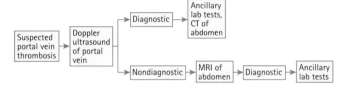

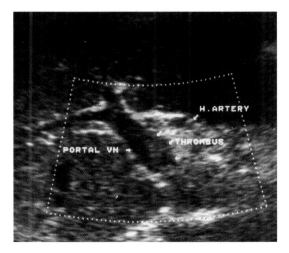

Figure 3-35 Portal venous thrombosis. Partial portal venous thrombosis is visible on B mode as echoreflective material on one side of the vein *(arrows)*. Doppler examination is always required to assess patency as some thrombi are of reduced echoreflectivity and may not be visible on B mode. *(From Grainger RG, Allison DJ, Adam A, Dixon AK, eds: Grainger & Allison's Diagnostic Radiology, ed 4, Churchill Livingstone, Philadelphia, 2001.)*

Diagnostic Imaging

Best Test(s)
• MRI of pituitary with gadolinium

Ancillary Tests
• CT of pituitary with contrast if MRI is contraindicated

Lab Evaluation

Best Test(s)
• Serum prolactin level

Ancillary Tests
• TRH stimulation (useful in equivocal cases); normal response is increase in serum prolactin level by 100% within 1 hour of TRH infusion; failure to increase is suggestive of pituitary lesion

Diagnostic Algorithm

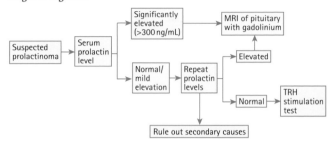

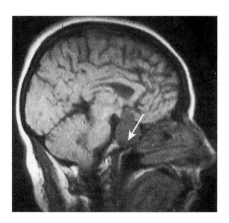

Figure 3-36 T1 Sagittal MRI depicting a large pituitary prolactinoma in a 13-year-old girl presenting with head-aches and galactorrhoea. *(From Grainger RG, Allison DJ, Adam A, Dixon AK, eds: Grainger & Allison's Diagnostic Radiology, ed 4, Churchill Livingstone, Philadelphia, 2001.)*

Diagnostic Imaging

Best Test(s)
• Transrectal ultrasound (useful to guide needle biopsy)

Ancillary Tests
• MRI of pelvis (useful to detect local spread and lymph node metastases)
• Bone scan (useful only for clinically suspected skeletal metastases)

Lab Evaluation

Best Test(s)
• Prostate biopsy

Ancillary Tests
• PSA
• Free PSA (higher free PSA in men with BPH vs. higher protein-bound PSA in men with prostate cancer)

Diagnostic Algorithm

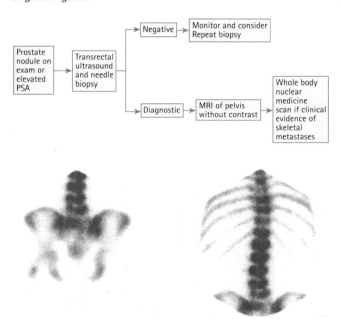

Figure 3-37 Technetium bone scan. Increased tracer activity is seen throughout the axial skeleton secondary to metastatic prostate cancer. *(From Hochberg MC, Silma AJ, Smolen JS, Weinblatt ME, Weisman MH, eds: Rheumatology, ed 3, St. Louis, Mosby, 2003.)*

Diagnostic Imaging

Best Test(s)
• None

Ancillary Tests
• Ultrasound of kidneys

Lab Evaluation

Best Test(s)
• 24-hour urine protein collection

Ancillary Tests
• Serum glucose, BUN, creatinine
• Urine protein IEP
• ANA; serum C3, C4
• Serum c-ANCA, p-ANCA
• Anti-GB membrane Ab
• HBsAg, HCV, HIV
• CBC

Diagnostic Algorithm

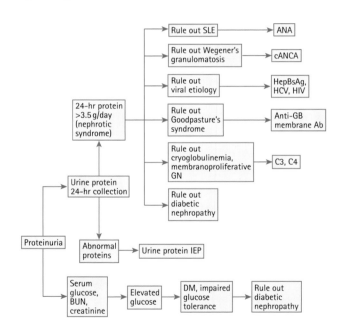

Diagnostic Imaging

Best Test(s)
• None

Ancillary Tests
• Chest radiograph
• CT of abdomen and chest with IV
  contrast

Lab Evaluation

Best Test(s)
• CBC with differential

Ancillary Tests
• ESR (nonspecific)
• FBS, BUN, creatinine
• ALT, AST, alkaline phosphatase,
  bilirubin
• TSH

Diagnostic Algorithm

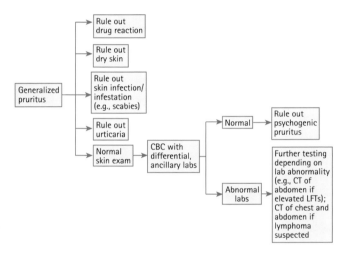

Diagnostic Imaging

Best Test(s)
• None

Ancillary Tests
• Abdominal plain film (flat plate and upright; useful in patients with abdominal pain or evidence of obstruction on exam)
• CT of abdomen

Lab Evaluation

Best Test(s)
• Stool test for *C. difficile* toxin assay (sensitivity 85%, specificity 100%)

Ancillary Tests
• CBC with differential

Diagnostic Algorithm

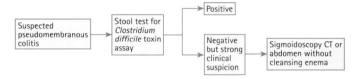

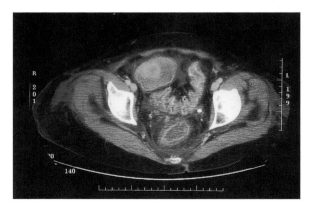

Figure 3-38 CT scan of the abdomen in a patient with fulminant Pseudomembromous colitis (PMC). The colonic and rectal walls are markedly thickened with fluid-filled colon and rectum. *(From Cohen J, Powderly WG: Infectious Diseases, ed 2, St. Louis, Mosby, 2004.)*

Diagnostic Imaging

Best Test(s)
• None

Ancillary Tests
• MRI of pituitary with gadolinium
• Pelvic ultrasound (females)
• Bone age (hand and wrist film)

Lab Evaluation

Best Test(s)
• FSH, LH

Ancillary Tests
• Prolactin
• Serum free testosterone
• GnRH
• Chromosomal karyotyping

Diagnostic Algorithm

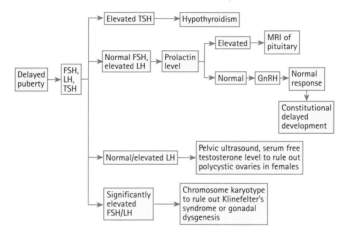

Diagnostic Imaging

Best Test(s)
• MRI of pituitary with gadolinium

Ancillary Tests
• CT of pituitary if MRI is contraindicated
• MRI or CT of adrenal glands (r/o neoplasm)
• Ultrasound of testicle in patient with unilateral testicular swelling

Lab Evaluation

Best Test(s)
• LH, FSH
• GnRH

Ancillary Tests
• hCG
• Serum testosterone (males)
• TSH
• DHEAS, D4 androstenedione
• Dexamethasone suppression test

Diagnostic Algorithm

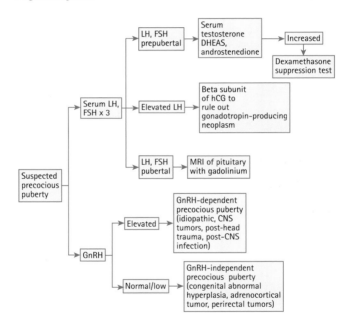

TABLE 3-3 Protocol for Investigation of Precocious Puberty

History, family history	
Exposure to environmental sex steroids	
Physical examination	Cutaneous lesions, e.g., neurofibromatosis, McCune-Albright syndrome
	CNS examination
Auxology	Pubertal staging (Tanner)
	Height, weight, height velocity
	Bone age
Hormone measurements	Testosterone/estradiol
	Luteinizing hormone/follicle-stimulating hormone
	Adrenal androgens (DHEA-S, androstenedione)
	17-hydroxyprogesterone + ACTH stimulation test hCG-ß
	Gonadotropin-releasing hormone test
Radiology	Pelvic ultrasound
	Magnetic resonance imaging of the hypothalamic-pituitary region
DNA analysis for known genetic disorders (testotoxicosis, McCune-Albright syndrome)	

DHEA-S, Dihydroepiandrosterone sulfate.
(From Besser CM, Thorner MO: *Comprehensive Clinical Endocrinology*, ed 3, St. Louis, Mosby, 2002.)

Diagnostic Imaging

Best Test(s)
- Spiral CT with IV contrast is best screening test to r/o PE in patients with baseline chest radiograph abnormalities

Ancillary Tests
- V/Q scan (when readily available, is useful as initial test in patients without baseline chest x-ray abnormalities)
- Pulmonary angiography gold standard but invasive and not readily available)
- Compressive Duplex ultrasonography of lower extremities (useful in patients with inconclusive lung scan or spiral CT and high clinical-suspicion)

Lab Evaluation

Best Test(s)
- D-Dimer by ELISA (normal D-dimer assay in patients with low probability of PE excludes diagnosis; normal D-dimer in patients with nondiagnostic lung scan, negative Doppler ultrasound of extremities, and low clinical suspicion excludes DVT)

Ancillary Tests
- ABGs (decreased PaO_2, $PaCO_2$, elevated pH)
- Alveolar-arterial (A-a) oxygen gradient; measure of the difference in oxygen concentration between alveoli and arterial blood; a normal A-a gradient

Diagnostic Algorithm

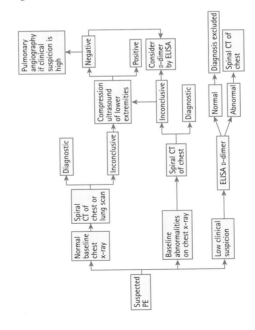

TABLE 3-4 Advantages and Limitations of Imaging Methods for Diagnosis of Pulmonary Embolism

Feature	Transthoracic Echocardiography	Lung Scanning	Pulmonary Angiography	Spiral CT Scanning
Widely available	+ + +	+ + +	+ +	+ +
Noninvasive	+ + +	+ +	−	+ +
Low interobserver variability	+ +	+ +	+ +	+ +
Well tolerated	+ + +	+ +	+	+ +
Detects massive PE	+ + +	+ +	+ + +	+ + +
Detects peripheral PE		+	+ + +	+ +
Low cost	+ + +	+ +	+	+

+ + +, Very good; + +, satisfactory; +, poor; −, does not apply.
From Crawford MH, DiMarco JP, Paulus WJ, eds: *Cardiology*, ed 2, St. Louis, Mosby, 2004.

176. Pulmonary Hypertension

Diagnostic Imaging

Best Test(s)
• Cardiac catheterization with direct measurement of pulmonary arterial pressure (useful for ruling out cardiac causes of pulmonary hypertension)

Ancillary Tests
• Chest radiograph (may reveal dilation of central arteries with rapid tapering of the distal vessels)
• Echocardiogram (to assess ventricular function and exclude significant valvular pathology)
• Spiral CT of chest if pulmonary embolism is suspected

Lab Evaluation

Best Test(s)
• None

Ancillary Tests
• CBC (erythrocytosis)
• ABGs (decreased Pao_2, decreased oxygen saturation)
• PFTs (r/o obstructive or restrictive lung disease)
• ECG (right ventricular hypertrophy)

Diagnostic Algorithm

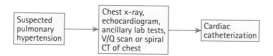

Suspected pulmonary hypertension → Chest x-ray, echocardiogram, ancillary lab tests, V/Q scan or spiral CT of chest → Cardiac catheterization

Diagnostic Imaging

Best Test(s)
• Spiral CT of chest without contrast

Ancillary Tests
• PET scan

Lab Evaluation

Best Test(s)
• Needle biopsy of nodule

Ancillary Tests
• None

Diagnostic Algorithm

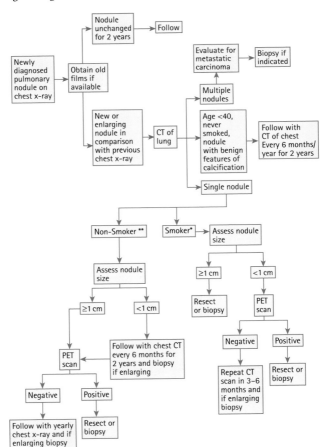

*Current or previous smoker
**Never smoked

Diagnostic Imaging

Best Test(s)
- None

Ancillary Tests
- Chest radiograph when collagen vascular disease or Wegener's granulomatosis is suspected
- Echocardiogram when endocarditis is suspected

Lab Evaluation

Best Test(s)
- Platelet count

Ancillary Tests
- CBC, peripheral blood smear, PT, PTT
- ANA (r/o vasculitis, collagen vascular disease)
- ALT, AST, creatinine
- Serum cryoglobulins (r/o mixed cryoglobulinemia)
- Serum protein IEP (r/o hyperglobulinemia)
- Blood culture × 2 (r/o SBE)
- c-ANCA (r/o Wegener's), p-ANCA (r/o vasculitis)

Diagnostic Algorithm

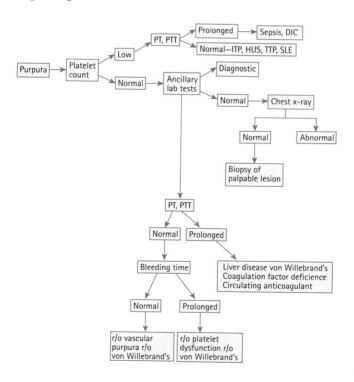

Diagnostic Imaging

Best Test(s)
• NONE

Ancillary Tests
• Radiograph of affected limb (r/o other cause of patient's symptoms)
• Three-phase radionuclide bone scan

Lab Evaluation

Best Test(s)
• None

Ancillary Tests
• CBC, ESR
• ANA
• FBS

Diagnostic Algorithm

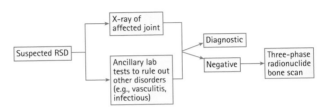

Diagnostic Imaging

Best Test(s)
• MRA of renal arteries

Ancillary Tests
• Ultrasound of kidneys
• Captopril renal scan if surgery is contemplated
• Angiography (diagnostic and can also be used for intervention [angioplasty, stent placement])

Lab Evaluation

Best Test(s)
• Selective renal vein renin measurement (gold standard but is invasive and expensive)

Ancillary Tests
• Serum creatinine, BUN, electrolytes
• Urinalysis

Diagnostic Algorithm

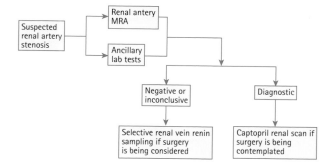

Diagnostic Imaging

Best Test(s)
• Renal ultrasound

Ancillary Tests
• Chest radiograph (r/o pleural effusion, pulmonary/renal syndromes [e.g., Goodpasture's, Wegener's])
• CT scan of kidneys without contrast (r/o suspected obstruction)

Lab Evaluation

Best Test(s)
• BUN/creatinine ratio (> 20:1 in prerenal and postrenal; < 2 0:1 in intrinsic renal failure)

Ancillary Tests
• Serum osmolality, urine osmolality
• Serum electrolytes, calcium, phosphate, uric acid, magnesium
• Calculate fractional excretion of sodium (FEna) = [Una/Pna/Ucreat/Pcreat × 100]; FEna < 1 in prerenal, > 1 in intrinsic renal failure

---

Diagnostic Algorithm

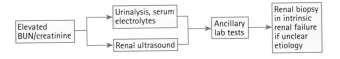

Diagnostic Imaging

Best Test(s)
• CT of kidneys with and without IV contrast

Ancillary Tests
• Renal ultrasound if cystic lesion
• MRI of kidneys when renal vein or caval thrombosis is suspected, or when CT is contraindicated
• IVP (role in evaluation of renal mass is questionable [lack of sensitivity and specificity, high radiation dose])

Lab Evaluation

Best Test(s)
• Urinalysis

Ancillary Tests
• Serum creatinine, calcium, albumin
• ESR (nonspecific)
• CBC

Diagnostic Algorithm

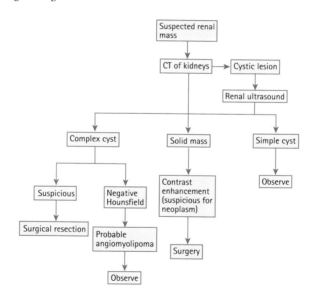

Diagnostic Imaging

Best Test(s)
• Renal angiography

Ancillary Tests
• Doppler ultrasound of abdomen (often initial study)
• MRI of abdomen
• CT of abdomen with contrast

Lab Evaluation

Best Test(s)
• None

Ancillary Tests
• Urinalysis
• Coagulopathy screen (PT, PTT, factor V leiden platelets, antithrombin III, protein C, protein S, lupus anticoagulant)
• Serum electrolytes, BUN, creatinine, ALT, AST, FBS

Diagnostic Algorithm

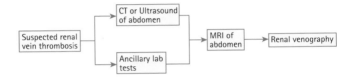

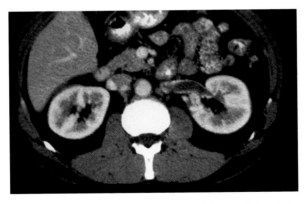

Figure 3-39 Renal vein thrombosis. CT scan showing left renal vein thrombosis (*Courtesty of Dr. S. Rankin. From Johnson RJ, Feehally J: Comprehensive Clinical Nephrology, ed 2, St. Louis, Mosby, 2000.*)

Diagnostic Imaging

Best Test(s)
• None

Ancillary Tests
• Chest radiograph

Lab Evaluation

Best Test(s)
• Serum electrolytes
• ABGs

Ancillary Tests
• BUN, creatinine

Diagnostic Algorithm

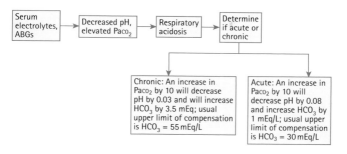

---

185. Respiratory Alkalosis

Diagnostic Imaging

Best Test(s)
• None

Ancillary Tests
• Chest radiograph

Lab Evaluation

Best Test(s)
• Serum electrolytes
• ABGs

Ancillary Tests
• BUN, creatinine

Diagnostic Algorithm

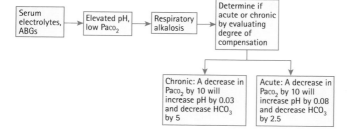

Diagnostic Imaging

Best Test(s)
- CT of soft tissues of neck with IV contrast

Ancillary Tests
- Lateral soft tissue radiograph of neck (often initial study)
- MRI of neck

Lab Evaluation

Best Test(s)
- None

Ancillary Tests
- CBC with differential
- Throat C&S
- Blood culture × 2

Diagnostic Algorithm

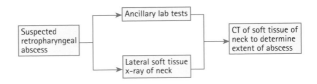

---

187.   Rhabdomyolysis

Diagnostic Imaging

Best Test(s)
- None

Ancillary Tests
- None

Lab Evaluation

Best Test(s)
- CPK with fractionation

Ancillary Tests
- Serum BUN, creatinine, electrolytes, calcium, phosphate, ALT, AST, uric acid
- CBC, urinalysis
- Serum and urine myoglobin levels

Diagnostic Algorithm

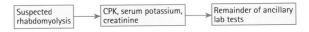

Diagnostic Imaging

Best Test(s)
• MRI of shoulder without contrast

Ancillary Tests
• Ultrasound of upper extremity may be used to diagnose suspected supraspinatus tear; major weakness in evaluating shoulder impingement is inability to visualize complete labrum; accuracy depends on skill of operator
• MRI arthrography (useful in shoulder instability for diagnosing labral tears)

Lab Evaluation

Best Test(s)
• None

Ancillary Tests
• None

Diagnostic Algorithm

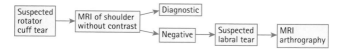

Suspected rotator cuff tear → *MRI of shoulder without contrast* → *Diagnostic*
→ *Negative* → *Suspected labral tear* → *MRI arthrography*

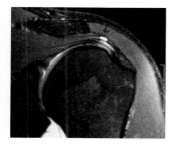

Figure 3-40 MRI of complex rotator cuff pathology. The image shows a partial articular surface rotator cuff tear along with a laminar defect and small cyst in the distal supraspinatus tendon. *(From Hochberg MC, Silma AJ, Smolen JS, Weinblatt ME, Weisman MH, eds: Rheumatology, ed 3, St. Louis, Mosby, 2003.)*

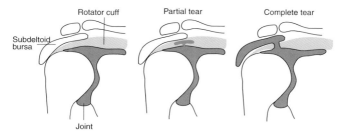

Figure 3-41 Rotator cuff tear. *(From Weissleder R, Wittenberg J, Harisinghani MG, Chen JW: Primer of Diagnostic Imaging, ed 4, St. Louis, Mosby, 2007.)*

Diagnostic Imaging

Best Test(s)
- Plain films of pelvis and AP lumbar spine

Ancillary Tests
- MRI of pelvis without contrast or nuclear medicine scan (only in selected cases)

Lab Evaluation

Best Test(s)
- None

Ancillary Tests
- CBC
- ESR (nonspecific)
- Serum calcium, alkaline phosphatase
- ANA

Diagnostic Algorithm

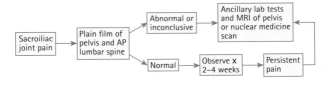

190.   Salivary Gland Neoplasm

Diagnostic Imaging

Best Test(s)
- CT of parotid gland with IV contrast

Ancillary Tests
- MRI of parotid gland (also an excellent diagnostic modality)
- MRI or CT sialography (useful for evaluation of salivary gland obstruction)
- Salivary gland ultrasound screening modality of choice when calculus is suspected)

Lab Evaluation

Best Test(s)
- Tissue diagnosis (biopsy)

Ancillary Tests
- Serum calcium, ALT, CBC

Diagnostic Algorithm

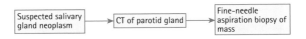

Diagnostic Imaging

Best Test(s)
• CT of chest with contrast

Ancillary Tests
• Chest radiograph (often reveals hilar and paratracheal adenopathy)

Lab Evaluation

Best Test(s)
• Biopsy of accessible tissue suspected of sarcoid involvement (e.g., lymph node, skin, conjunctiva)

Ancillary Tests
• CBC, ESR
• ALT, AST, serum calcium
• Serum ACE level
• PFTs

Diagnostic Algorithm

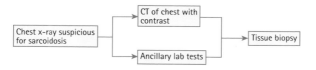

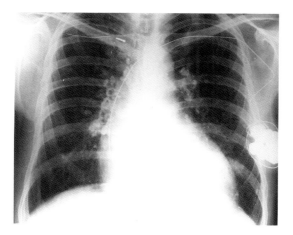

Figure 3-42 "Eggshell" calcification in sarcoidosis. There is extensive calcification of the hilar and mediastinal lymph nodes; the calcification has a peripheral (eggshell) configuration, particularly in lymph nodes at the right hilum. Cardiac involvement necessitated the pacemaker. *(From Grainger RG, Allison DJ, Adam A, Dixon AK, eds: Grainger & Allison's Diagnostic Radiology, ed 4, Churchill Livingstone, Philadelphia, 2001.)*

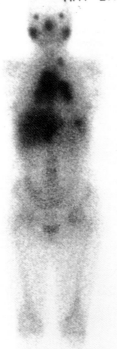

Figure 3-43 Abnormal gallium scan in sarcoidosis. The scan shows uptake in the lacrimal, parotid, and salivary glands (panda sign), as well as mediastinal lymph nodes (lambda sign) and lungs. *(From Hochberg MC, Silma AJ, Smolen JS, Weinblatt ME, Weisman MH, eds: Rheumatology, ed 3, St. Louis, Mosby, 2003.)*

Diagnostic Imaging

Best Test(s)
• Ultrasound of scrotum

Ancillary Tests
• MRI of pelvis with and without contrast for staging of neoplasm

Lab Evaluation

Best Test(s)
• None

Ancillary Tests
• Urinalysis
• CBC with differential
• Serum alpha-fetoprotein
• Serum hCG

Diagnostic Algorithm

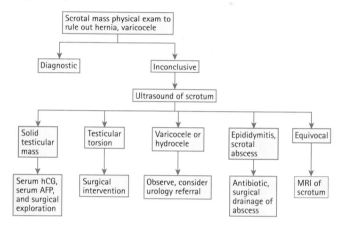

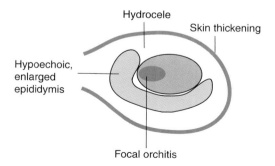

Figure 3-44 Scrotal mass. *(From Weissleder R, Wittenberg J, Harisinghani MG, Chen JW: Primer of Diagnostic Imaging, ed 4, St. Louis, Mosby, 2007.)*

Diagnostic Imaging

Best Test(s)
- MRI of brain

Ancillary Tests
- CT of brain with and without contrast if MRI is contraindicated or hemorrhage is suspected

Lab Evaluation

Best Test(s)
- None

Ancillary Tests
- Serum glucose, electrolytes
- CBC
- Toxicology screen

Diagnostic Algorithm

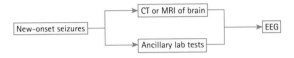

---

194.   SIADH

Diagnostic Imaging

Best Test(s)
- None

Ancillary Tests
- Chest radiograph (r/o neoplasm, infectious process)
- MRI of brain (r/o CNS lesion)

Lab Evaluation

Best Test(s)
- Serum electrolytes, osmolality
- Urine sodium, urine osmolality
- BUN, creatinine

Ancillary Tests
- Serum uric acid (decreased)
- TSH
- Serum cortisol

Diagnostic Algorithm

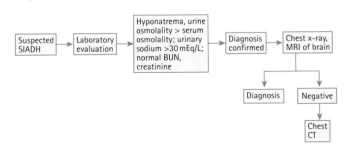

Diagnostic Imaging

Best Test(s)
• Sialography

Ancillary Tests
• CT scan of salivary gland if neoplasm is suspected

Lab Evaluation

Best Test(s)
• None

Ancillary Tests
• Serum calcium, phosphate
• CBC

Diagnostic Algorithm

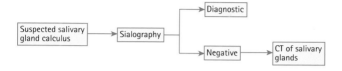

196. Sinusitis

Diagnostic Imaging

Best Test(s)
• Coronal CT of sinuses without contrast (generally reserved for complicated sinusitis or to define anatomy before surgery)

Ancillary Tests
• Radiograph of sinuses (of limited use in diagnosis)
• MRI of sinuses (cannot define anatomy as well as CT; may be useful only for differentiating soft tissue structures [e.g., neoplasm, fungal infection])

Lab Evaluation

Best Test(s)
• Sinus aspiration and culture

Ancillary Tests
• CBC with differential

Diagnostic Algorithm

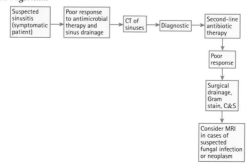

Diagnostic Imaging

Best Test(s)
- Plain film of abdomen; AP is best initial study

Ancillary Tests
- CT of abdomen and pelvis with IV contrast (will confirm obstruction)
- Small-bowel series (may be necessary for defining level of obstruction)

Lab Evaluation

Best Test(s)
- None

Ancillary Tests
- CBC with differential
- Serum electrolytes, BUN, creatinine
- ALT, AST, alkaline phosphatase
- Urinalysis, urine C&S
- Glucose, amylase

Diagnostic Algorithm

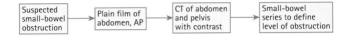

| Suspected small-bowel obstruction | → | Plain film of abdomen, AP | → | CT of abdomen and pelvis with contrast | → | Small-bowel series to define level of obstruction |

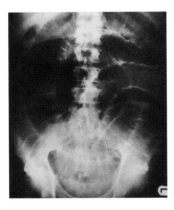

Figure 3-45 Small-bowel obstruction. Supine very distended small bowel identified by its central position, multiple loops, and valulae conniventes. Nondistended ascending colon can be identified. *(From Grainger RG, Allison DJ, Adam A, Dixon AK, eds: Grainger & Allison's Diagnostic Radiology, ed 4, Churchill Livingstone, Philadelphia, 2001.)*

Diagnostic Imaging

Best Test(s)
• MRI with gadolinium of spinal cord

Ancillary Tests
• CT with myelography (more sensitive for cord compression)

Lab Evaluation

Best Test(s)
• Gram stain and C&S of abscess content

Ancillary Tests
• CBC with differential
• Blood culture × 2
• ESR

Diagnostic Algorithm

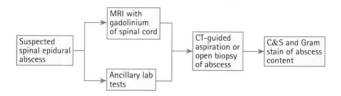

---

199. Spinal Stenosis

Diagnostic Imaging

Best Test(s)
• MRI of spine (sensitivity 80%-90%, specificity 95%)

Ancillary Tests
• CT of spine (sensitivity 75%-85%, specificity 80%) if MRI is contraindicated

Lab Evaluation

Best Test(s)
• None

Ancillary Tests
• None

Diagnostic Algorithm

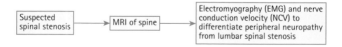

Diagnostic Imaging

Best Test(s)
• CT of abdomen

Ancillary Tests
• Ultrasound of abdomen if CT is contraindicated
• Echocardiography if CHF or SBE is suspected

Lab Evaluation

Best Test(s)
• CBC with differential

Ancillary Tests
• Viral titers (EB, CMV)
• ALT, AST, bilirubin, albumin, INR
• ESR, RF, ANA
• Blood culture × 2 if splenic abscess is suspected

Diagnostic Algorithm

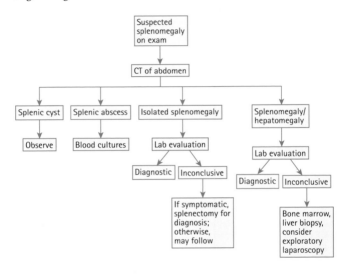

Diagnostic Imaging

Best Test(s)
• CT of brain without contrast

Ancillary Tests
• Cerebral angiography

Lab Evaluation

Best Test(s)
• None

Ancillary Tests
• PT, PTT, platelet count
• CBC

Diagnostic Algorithm

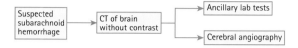

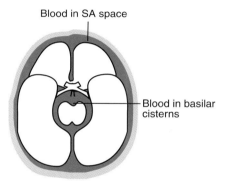

Figure 3-46 Subarachnoid hemorrhage.
(From Weissleder R, Wittenberg J, Harisinghani MG, Chen JW: Primer of Diagnostic Imaging, ed 4, St. Louis, Mosby, 2007.)

Diagnostic Imaging

Best Test(s)
• Arteriography of subclavian and
  vertebral innominate arteries

Ancillary Tests
• Doppler sonography of vertebral,
  subclavian, and innominate arteries
  (best initial screening test)

Lab Evaluation

Best Test(s)
• None

Ancillary Tests
• Lipid panel
• FBS
• ANA, ESR

Diagnostic Algorithm

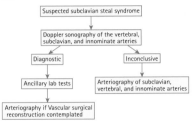

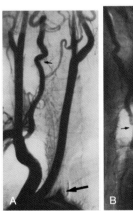
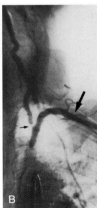

Figure 3-47 Subclavian steal: arch aortogram. **A,** Left
anterior oblique projection, arterial phase: proximal
occlusion of the left subclavian artery *(arrow)*. Note ir-
regularity and tortuosity of right vertebral artery related
to degenerative changes in the cervical vertebrae *(small
arrow)*. **B,** Right anterior oblique projection late phase
of aortogram; the distal segment of the left subclavian
artery *(arrow)* fills via retrograde flow in the left vertebral artery, despite this vessel being almost completely
obstructed at its origin *(small arrow)*. *(From Grainger
RG, Allison DJ, Adam A, Dixon AK, eds: Grainger &
Allison's Diagnostic Radiology, ed 4, Churchill
Livingstone, Philadelphia, 2001.)*

Diagnostic Imaging

Best Test(s)
• CT of brain without contrast

Ancillary Tests
• None

Lab Evaluation

Best Test(s)
• None

Ancillary Tests
• PT, PTT, platelet count
• CBC

Diagnostic Algorithm

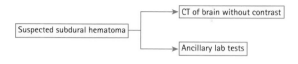

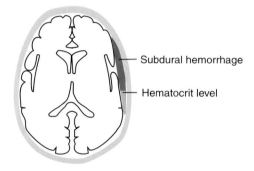

Figure 3-48 Subdural hematoma. *(From Weissleder R, Wittenberg J, Harisinghani MG, Chen JW: Primer of Diagnostic Imaging, ed 4, St. Louis, Mosby, 2007.)*

Diagnostic Imaging

Best Test(s)
• Venography of superior vena cava

Ancillary Tests
• CT of chest

Lab Evaluation

Best Test(s)
• None

Ancillary Tests
• Tissue biopsy of mediastinal mass
  (e.g., lymphoma, lung carcinoma)
  compressing superior vena cava

Diagnostic Algorithm

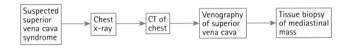

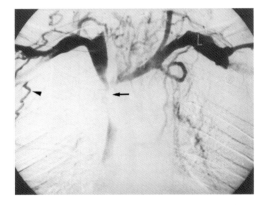

Figure 3-49 Upper limb venography. Bilateral arm venography
reveals obstruction of the SVC by tumor in the mediastinum
(arrow). This was a case of SVC syndrome secondary to lung
carcinoma metastatic disease. Note the collateral venous channels
that have opened up *(arrowhead)*. *(From Grainger RG, Allison
DJ, Adam A, Dixon AK, eds: Grainger & Allison's Diagnostic
Radiology, ed 4, Churchill Livingstone, Philadelphia, 2001.)*

Diagnostic Imaging

Best Test(s)
- None; diagnostic imaging should be guided by history and physical exam

Ancillary Tests
- Echocardiography (useful in patients with a heart murmur to r/o aortic stenosis, hypertrophic cardiomyopathy, or atrial myxoma)
- CT of head and EEG if seizure is suspected
- Spiral CT of chest or V/Q scan if PE is suspected

Lab Evaluation

Best Test(s)
- None

Ancillary Tests
- Routine blood tests (rarely yield diagnostically useful information and should be done only when specifically suggested by history and physical exam)
- Serum pregnancy test (should be considered in women of childbearing age)
- CBC, electrolytes, BUN, creatinine
- Serum calcium, magnesium
- ABGs
- ECG
- Cardiac troponins, isoenzymes if history of chest pain before syncope
- Toxicology screen in selected patients
- Cardiac stress test
- Electrophysiologic (EPS) studies

Diagnostic Algorithm

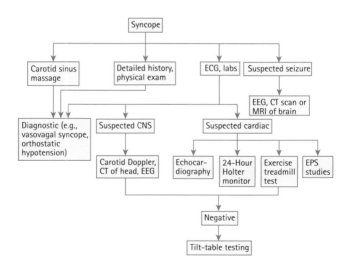

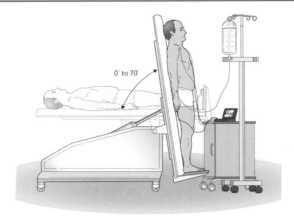

Figure 3-50 A 70-degree tilt test using a motorized table with a footplate. Not illustrated are ECG leads for monitoring and a cuff or continuous blood pressure monitor. *(From Crawford MH, DiMarco JP, Paulus WJ, eds: Cardiology, ed 2, St. Louis, Mosby, 2004.)*

206. Temporal (Giant Cell) Arteritis

Diagnostic Imaging

Best Test(s)
• NONE

Ancillary Tests
• Chest radiograph and ultrasound of abdominal aorta in documented temporal arteritis (increased risk of aneurysm)
• Color duplex arteriography of temporal artery (positive test reveals a dark halo caused by edema of artery wall)

Lab Evaluation

Best Test(s)
• Temporal artery biopsy
• ESR

Ancillary Tests
• CBC, ALT, alkaline phosphatase

Diagnostic Algorithm

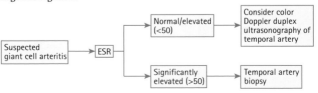

Diagnostic Imaging

Best Test(s)
• MRI of TMJ without contrast

Ancillary Tests
• CT scan of TMJ without contrast
(if MRI is contraindicated; useful for
diagnosis of meniscal and osseous
derangement of TMJ)

Lab Evaluation

Best Test(s)
• None

Ancillary Tests
• None

Diagnostic Algorithm

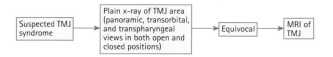

---

208. Testicular Neoplasm

Diagnostic Imaging

Best Test(s)
• Ultrasound of testicle (best screening
test)

Ancillary Tests
• CT of chest, abdomen, and pelvis if
diagnosis is confirmed

Lab Evaluation

Best Test(s)
• Serum hCG (elevated)
• Serum alpha-fetoprotein (elevated)

Ancillary Tests
• Serum LDH

Diagnostic Algorithm

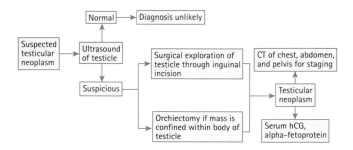

Diagnostic Imaging

Best Test(s)
• Doppler ultrasound of testicle (Doppler flowmetry)

Ancillary Tests
• Tc-99m testicular scan also an excellent modality for evaluating blood flow to testicle (absence of blood flow centrally to testicle indicates torsion)

Lab Evaluation

Best Test(s)
• None

Ancillary Tests
• None

Diagnostic Algorithm

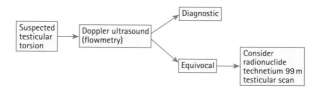

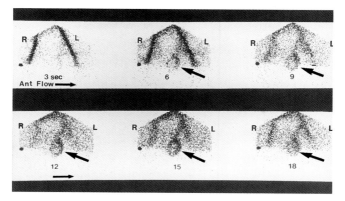

Figure 3-51 Testicular torsion. Evaluation of blood flow to the testicle has been done by giving an intravenous bolus of radioactive material. The right and left iliac vessels are clearly identified, and sequential images are obtained every 3 seconds. Here increased flow is seen to the rim of the left testicle *(arrows)*, and there is no blood flow centrally. This is the appearance of a testicular torsion in which the torsion has been present for more than approximately 24 hours. *(From Mettler FA, Guibertau MJ, Voss CM, Urbina CE: Primary Care Radiology, Philadelphia, WB Saunders, 2000.)*

Diagnostic Imaging

Best Test(s)
• Arteriography or venography when vascular pathology is suspected clinically

Ancillary Tests
• Chest radiograph (r/o cervical rib)
• X-ray of cervical spine (r/o cervical disk disease)
• CT of chest (r/o lung neoplasm)

Lab Evaluation

Best Test(s)
• None

Ancillary Tests
• EMG, nerve conduction studies

Diagnostic Algorithm

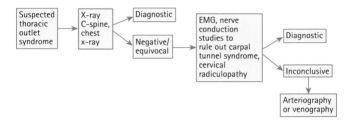

Diagnostic Imaging

Best Test(s)
• None

Ancillary Tests
• CT of abdomen if splenomegaly is present

Lab Evaluation

Best Test(s)
• Bone marrow exam

Ancillary Tests
• CBC, PT, PTT
• LDH
• HIV, ANA
• Antiplatelet Ab
• D-dimer
• Coombs' test

Diagnostic Algorithm

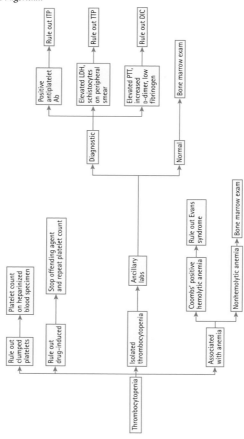

Diagnostic Imaging

Best Test(s)
• None

Ancillary Tests
• CT of chest and abdomen

Lab Evaluation

Best Test(s)
• Bone marrow exam

Ancillary Tests
• CBC
• Reticulocyte count
• Stool for occult blood × 3
• Serum ferritin, TIBC, iron

Diagnostic Algorithm

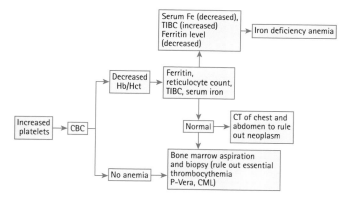

Diagnostic Imaging

Best Test(s)
- Thyroid ultrasound to evaluate size and composition of nodule (solid vs. cystic)

Ancillary Tests
- Thyroid scan with Tc-99m classifies nodule as hyperfunctioning [hot], normally functioning [warm], or nonfunctioning [cold]; thyroid scan can also be performed with iodine)

Lab Evaluation

Best Test(s)
- Fine-needle aspiration biopsy (FNAB)

Ancillary Tests
- TSH, free T_4
- Antimicrosomal Ab
- Serum calcium
- Serum thyroglobulin level in patients with confirmed thyroid carcinoma

Diagnostic Algorithm

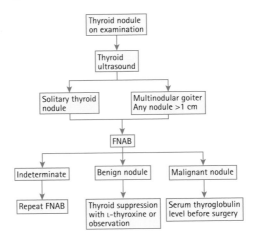

Diagnostic Imaging

Best Test(s)
- 24-hour RAIU scan (useful in distinguishing Graves' disease [increased RAIU] from thyroiditis [normal/low RAIU])

Ancillary Tests
- Thyroid ultrasound

Lab Evaluation

Best Test(s)
- None

Ancillary Tests
- TSH, free T_4
- CBC with differential (leukocytosis with left shift occurs with subacute and suppurative thyroiditis)
- Antimicrosomal AB (detected in > 90% of patients with Hashimoto's thyroiditis)
- Serum thyroglobulin level (increased in patients with autoimmune lymphocytic thyroiditis)

Diagnostic Algorithm

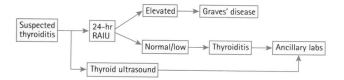

Diagnostic Imaging

Best Test(s)
• None

Ancillary Tests
• Carotid Doppler ultrasound
• MRI of brain and auditory canals
• Brain MRA

Lab Evaluation

Best Test(s)
• None

Ancillary Tests
• CBC
• Lipid panel

Diagnostic Algorithm

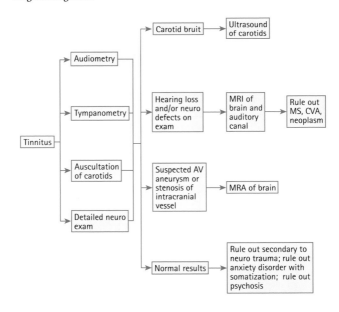

Diagnostic Imaging

Best Test(s)
• Carotid Doppler (to identify carotid stenosis)

Ancillary Tests
• CT of head without contrast (r/o hemorrhage or subdural hematoma)
• Echocardiography (if cardiac source is suspected)
• Brain MRA if posterior circulation TIA is suspected

Lab Evaluation

Best Test(s)
• None

Ancillary Tests
• PT, PTT, platelet count
• Lipid panel, FBS
• ESR

Diagnostic Algorithm

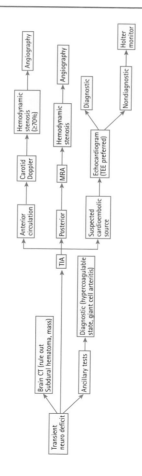

Diagnostic Imaging

Best Test(s)
- MRI of head and neck with IV contrast

Ancillary Tests
- CT scan with thin posterior fossa cuts if MRI is contraindicated; exam is limited

Lab Evaluation

Best Test(s)
- None

Ancillary Tests
- ESR
- CBC with differential

Diagnostic Algorithm

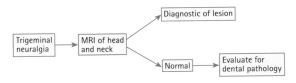

Diagnostic Imaging

Best Test(s)
• None

Ancillary Tests
• None

Lab Evaluation

Best Test(s)
• Gram stain of exudate
• Gonorrhea culture on Thayer-Martin medium or PCR assay
• Culture for *C. trachomatis* or PCR assay

Ancillary Tests
• Wet mount for *Trichomonas*
• HIV, VDRL

Diagnostic Algorithm

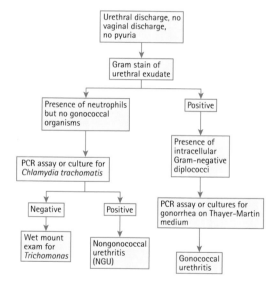

Diagnostic Imaging

Best Test(s)
- Noncontrast helical CT of urinary tract

Ancillary Tests
- Renal sonogram
- IVP (demonstrates size and location of calculus)
- Plain film of abdomen (can identify radiopaque stones [e.g., calcium])

Lab Evaluation

Best Test(s)
- Urinalysis

Ancillary Tests
- Chemical analysis of recovered stone
- Serum calcium, phosphate, uric acid, BUN, creatinine
- Urine C&S
- 4-hour urine for calcium in patients with calcium stones

Diagnostic Algorithm

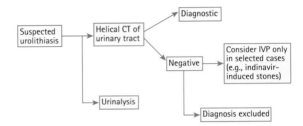

Diagnostic Imaging

Best Test(s)
• None

Ancillary Tests
• Chest radiograph

Lab Evaluation

Best Test(s)
• None

Ancillary Tests
• CBC with differential
• ANA
• Hepatitis screen
• ALT, Monospot
• Thyroid antibodies
• Stool for ova and parasites

Diagnostic Algorithm

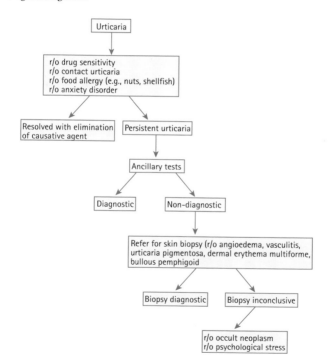

Diagnostic Imaging

Best Test(s)
• Obstetric ultrasound

Ancillary Tests
• None

Lab Evaluation

Best Test(s)
• Serum quantitative hCG

Ancillary Tests
• CBC, platelet count
• PT, PTT

Diagnostic Algorithm

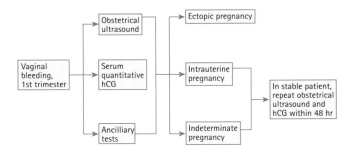

Diagnostic Imaging

Best Test(s)
• None

Ancillary Tests
• None

Lab Evaluation

Best Test(s)
• Wet mount and KOH preparation

Ancillary Tests
• Gonorrhea culture on Thayer-Martin medium
• Culture for *C. trachomatis*
• HIV
• PCR assay for gonosshea

Diagnostic Algorithm

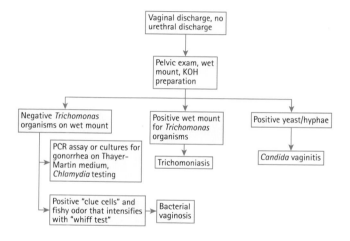

Diagnostic Imaging

Best Test(s)
• MRI of brain

Ancillary Tests
• MRA of posterior circulation
  (CT of cerebellopontine region if
  MRI is contraindicated)

Lab Evaluation

Best Test(s)
• None

Ancillary Tests
• CBC with differential
• Serum glucose, creatinine, ALT,
  electrolytes

Diagnostic Algorithm

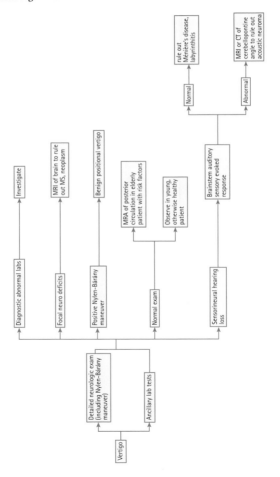

Diagnostic Imaging

Best Test(s)
• None

Ancillary Tests
• None

Lab Evaluation

Best Test(s)
• Hepatitis panel (should include HBsAg, anti-HBc IgM, anti-HAV IgM, anti-HCV)

Ancillary Tests
• ALT, AST
• Alkaline phosphatase, bilirubin, PT
• ANA, anti–smooth muscle antibody, antimitochondrial antibody if autoimmune hepatitis is suspected

Diagnostic Algorithm

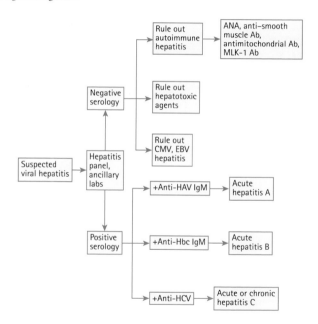

Diagnostic Imaging

Best Test(s)
• None

Ancillary Tests
• None

Lab Evaluation

Best Test(s)
• von Willebrand's factor (decreased)
• Decreased or absent platelet aggregation when ristocetin is added to patient's platelet-rich plasma
• Bleeding time (increased) or platelet function assay (PFA)
• Prolonged PTT

Ancillary Tests
• Factor VIII coagulant activity (decreased)
• Platelet count (normal)
• Platelet aggregation (normal)
• CBC

Diagnostic Algorithm

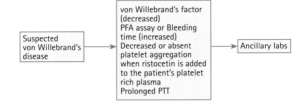

Diagnostic Imaging

Best Test(s)
• None

Ancillary Tests
• Chest radiograph (r/o pulmonary involvement)

Lab Evaluation

Best Test(s)
• Serum protein electrophoresis (reveals homogeneous M spike)
• IEP

Ancillary Tests
• CBC (anemia)
• ESR (increased due to rouleaux formation)
• Urine protein IEP (monoclonal light chains, usually kappa)
• Bone marrow biopsy
• Serum cryoglobulins
• Serum viscosity (elevated)

Diagnostic Algorithm

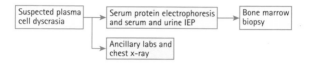

Diagnostic Imaging

Best Test(s)
- Chest radiograph (may reveal bilateral multiple nodules, cavitated mass lesions, pleural effusion)

Ancillary Tests
- Ultrasound of kidneys
- CT of sinuses and chest

Lab Evaluation

Best Test(s)
- Biopsy of affected organ (e.g., lung, nasopharynx)

Ancillary Tests
- Serum c-ANCA level
- Urinalysis (hematuria, RBC casts, proteinuria)
- CBC (anemia, leukocytosis)
- BUN, creatinine (increased)
- ESR (increased)

Diagnostic Algorithm

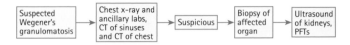

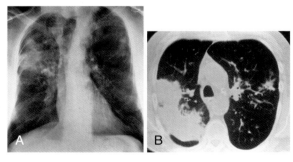

Figure 3-52 Wegener's granulomatosis. **A,** Chest radiograph showing bilateral patch air-space opacities; there is no evidence of caviation. **B,** CT through the upper zones with multifocal regions of dense parenchymal opacification.
(From Grainger RG, Allison DJ, Adam A, Dixon AK, eds: Grainger & Allison's Diagnostic Radiology, ed 4, Churchill Livingstone, Philadelphia, 2001.)

Diagnostic Imaging

Best Test(s)
• None

Ancillary Tests
• Chest radiograph
• Ultrasound of abdomen if cirrhosis or nephrosis suspected

Lab Evaluation

Best Test(s)
• TSH

Ancillary Tests
• FBS, BUN, creatinine, ALT
• Urinalysis
• Serum dehydroepiandrosterone level

Diagnostic Algorithm

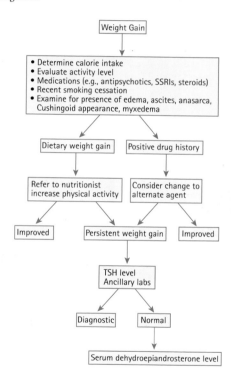

Diagnostic Imaging

Best Test(s)
• None

Ancillary Tests
• Chest radiograph

Lab Evaluation

Best Test(s)
• TSH, free T$_4$

Ancillary Tests
• CBC, glucose
• ESR (nonspecific)
• ALT, creatinine, serum albumin
• Urinalysis

Diagnostic Algorithm

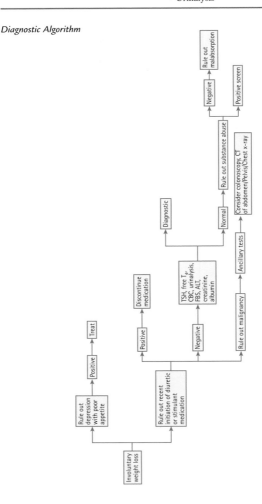

Diagnostic Imaging

Best Test(s)
• None

Ancillary Tests
• CT of liver in equivocal cases

Lab Evaluation

Best Test(s)
• Serum ceruloplasmin level (decreased)
• Serum copper level (decreased)
• 24-hour urinary copper excretion (increased)

Ancillary Tests
• CBC, bilirubin, reticulocyte count, haptoglobin if hemolytic anemia is suspected
• ALT, AST (increased)
• Liver biopsy with demonstration of elevated hepatic copper content (> 250 µg/g dry weight; normal is < 50 µg/g)
• Serum uric acid (decreased), phosphate (decreased)
• Urinalysis (hematuria)

Diagnostic Algorithm

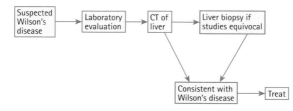

Diagnostic Imaging

Best Test(s)
• None

Ancillary Tests
• CT or MRI of abdomen with IV contrast
• Selective celiac arteriography for gastrinoma
• Octreotide nuclear medicine scan can be used for localization

Lab Evaluation

Best Test(s)
• Fasting serum gastrin level (>150 pg/ml)

Ancillary Tests
• Provocative gastrin level tests (secretin stimulation, calcium stimulation
• ALT, AST

Diagnostic Algorithm

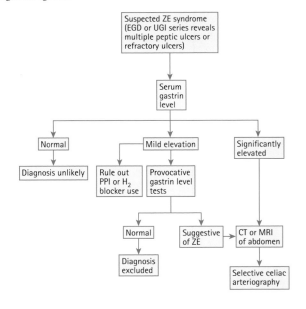

REFERENCES

1. Abeloff MD: *Clinical Oncology*, ed 2, New York, Churchill Livingstone, 2000.
2. Andreoli TE, ed: *Cecil Essentials of Medicine*, ed 4, Philadelphia, WB Saunders, 1997.
3. Carlson KJ, et al: *Primary Care of Women*, ed 2, St. Louis, Mosby, 2002.
4. Feldman M, et al: *Sleisenger and Fordtran's Gastrointestinal and Liver Diseases: Pathophysiology/Diagnosis/Management*, ed 6, Philadelphia, WB Saunders, 1998.
5. Gay SB, Woodcock RJ: *Radiology Recall,* Philadelphia, Lippincott Williams & Wilkins, 2000.
6. Goldman L, Ausiello D, eds: *Cecil Textbook of Medicine*, ed 22, Philadelphia, WB Saunders, 2004.
7. Greene HL, Johnson WP, Lemcke D, eds: *Decision Making in Medicine*, ed 2, St. Louis, Mosby, 1998.
8. Healey PM: *Common Medical Diagnosis: An Algorithmic Approach*, ed 3, Philadelphia, WB Saunders, 2000.
9. Henry JB, ed: *Clinical Diagnosis and Management by Laboratory Methods*, ed 20, Philadelphia, WB Saunders, 2001.
10. Kassirer J, ed: *Current Therapy in Adult Medicine*, ed 4, St. Louis, Mosby, 1998.
11. Marx JA, ed: *Rosen's Emergency Medicine*, St. Louis, Mosby, 2002.
12. Mettler FA, et al: *Primary Care Radiology*. Philadelphia, WB Saunders, 2000.
13. Moore WT, Eastman RC: *Diagnostic Endocrinology*, ed 2, St. Louis, Mosby, 1996.
14. Noble J: *Primary Care Medicine*, ed 3, St. Louis, Mosby, 2001.
15. Nseyo UO (ed): *Urology for Primary Care Physicians*, Philadelphia, WB Saunders, 1999.
16. Orrison WW, et al: *Pocket Medical Imaging Consultant*, Houston, HealthHelp, 2002.
17. Rakel RE, ed: *Principles of Family Practice*, ed 6, Philadelphia, WB Saunders, 2002.
18. Stein JH, ed: *Internal Medicine*, ed 5, St. Louis, Mosby, 1998.

INDEX

References are to pages. Pages followed by an "f" indicate figures; "t," tables.